Instructor's Resource Manual with Test Bank and PowerPoint Lecture CD-ROM

Tappan's Handbook of Healing Massage Techniques

Classic, Holistic, and Emerging Methods

Fourth Edition

Patricia J. Benjamin, PhD
Licensed Massage Therapist, Illinois

Frances M. Tappan, PT, EdD
Formerly of the University of Connecticut
Storrs, Connecticut

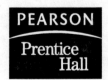

PEARSON
Prentice
Hall

Upper Saddle River, New Jersey

Notice: The authors and the publisher of this volume have taken care that the information and technical recommendations contained herein are based on research and expert consultation, and are accurate and compatible with the standards generally accepted at the time of publication. Nevertheless, as new information becomes available, changes in clinical and technical practices becomes necessary. The reader is advised to carefully consult manufacturers' instructions and information material for all supplies and equipment before use, and to consult with a healthcare professional as necessary. This advice is espcially important when using new supplies or equipment for clinical purposes. The authors and publisher disclaim all responsibility for any liability, loss, injury, or damage incurred as a consequence, directly or indirectly, of the use and application of any of the contents of this volume.

Copyright © 2005 by Pearson Education, Inc., Upper Saddle River, New Jersey, 07458.

Pearson Prentice Hall. All rights reserved. Printed in the United States of America. This publication is protected by Copyright and permission should be obtained from the publisher prior to any prohibited reproduction, storage in a retrieval system, or transmission in any form or by any means, electronic, mechanical, photocopying, recording, or likewise. For information regarding permission(s), write to: Rights and Permissions Department.

Pearson Prentice Hall™ is a trademark of Pearson Education, Inc.
Pearson® is a registered trademark of Pearson plc
Prentice Hall® is a registered trademark of Pearson Education, Inc.

Pearson Education, Ltd., *London*
Pearson Education Australia Pty. Limited, *Sydney*
Pearson Education Singapore, Pte. Ltd.
Pearson Education North Asia Ltd., *Hong Kong*
Pearson Education Canada, Ltd., *Toronto*

Pearson Educaçion de Mexico, S.A. de C.V.
Pearson Education—Japan, *Tokyo*
Pearson Education Malaysia, Pte. Ltd.
Pearson Education, Upper Saddle River, *New Jersey*

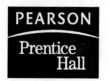

10 9 8 7 6 5 4 3 2 1
ISBN 0-13-111140-X

Contents

Preface

With its fourth edition, *Tappan's Handbook of Healing Massage Techniques* has been updated and redesigned to meet the educational needs of students and teachers. Along with new educational features in the book itself, this *Instructor's Resource Manual* provides teachers with the tools they need to plan courses, units, and individual lectures. The extensive text bank can serve as a base for evaluating students' knowledge and as preparation for licensing and certification examinations.

CD-ROM video that accompanies *Tappan's Handbook of Healing Massage Techniques* provides demonstrations of massage techniques and good body mechanics. It can be used in class to illustrate lectures or for demonstration in hands-on practice classes. It can be assigned as homework prior to class and for review as students practice outside of scheduled class time.

The *Instructor's Resource Manual* is printed on perforated paper with three-ring punch holes so that you can remove sections and use as needed to prepare for lessons. In addition, the contents are available on the accompanying CD using PowerPoint® software that allows teachers to modify the information electronically.

SUMMARY OF EDUCATIONAL FEATURES
IN *TAPPAN'S HANDBOOK OF HEALING MASSAGE TECHNIQUES*
AND THE ACCOMPANYING *INSTRUCTOR'S RESOURCE MANUAL*

Tappan's Handbook of Healing Massage Techniques
    Detailed Table of Contents
    List of Illustrations and Tables
    Chapters
        Learning Outcomes
        Key Terms and Concepts
        References
        Additional Resources (e.g., books, videos, Web sites)
        Study Guide (e.g., learning activities and fill-in-the blanks test)
    Appendices
        Massage and Bodywork Comparison Chart
        Organizations and Publications
        Massage Licensing Laws
        Performance Evaluation Forms
        Health History Forms
    Glossary
    Index
Instructor's Resource Manual
    Use of *Instructor's Resource Manual* for Planning
    Course Syllabi
    Lecture Outlines
    Suggested Classroom Activities
    Test Bank—Chapter by Chapter
    CD-ROM Video Segments Questions & Answers

**HOW TO BEST USE THE *INSTRUCTOR'S RESOURCE MANUAL*
WITH *TAPPAN'S HANDBOOK OF HEALING MASSAGE TECHNIQUES*
AND THE CD-ROM VIDEO**

Together *Tappan's Handbook of Healing Massage Techniques*, the CD-ROM video, and the *Instructor's Resource Manual* provide the curriculum coordinator and instructors the tools they need to develop comprehensive, informative, and exciting lessons for students of massage therapy.

PLANNING COURSES

- Choose the course syllabus from the *Instructor's Resource Manual* that most closely matches the course or unit you are planning. Modify topics, schedule, and evaluation as needed to fit your situation.

PLANNING LESSONS

- Determine the learning outcomes and key terms and concepts for the lesson using information at the beginning of the chapters in *Tappan's Handbook of Healing Massage Techniques*.

- Find additional resources (e.g., books, Web sites, and instructional videos) at the end of the chapters in *Tappan's Handbook of Healing Massage Techniques*.

- Review the *Tappan's Handbook of Healing Massage Techniques* CD-ROM video for segments relevant to the class topics. Prepare for use during class or as a preclass homework assignment.

- Integrate suggested classroom activities found in the *Instructor's Resource Manual* or exercises from the chapter *study guides* in *Tappan's Handbook of Healing Massage Techniques*.

- Determine student reading assignments matching lecture topics to information in the relevant *Tappan's Handbook of Healing Massage Techniques* chapter and the CD-ROM video.

PLANNING LECTURES

- Use the lecture outline from the *Instructor's Resource Manual* as it is presented, or modify as desired.*

- Choose suggested classroom activities from the *Instructor's Resource Manual* to enhance the lecture.

- Use references and additional resources listed at the end of each chapter in *Tappan's Handbook of Healing Massage Techniques* for further information on specific topics.

- Choose a segment from the *Tappan's Handbook of Healing Massage Techniques* CD-ROM video to show during lecture for illustration.

ENHANCE LEARNING

- Use the learning activities in the study guides at the end of each chapter in *Tappan's Handbook of Healing Massage Techniques* as in-class or homework assignments.

- Assign the fill-in-the-blanks study outlines at the end of the chapters in *Tappan's Handbook of Healing Massage Techniques* as homework to reinforce recall of the main ideas in each chapter or as preparation for an upcoming class.

- Assign the learning activities for greater understanding from the study guide at the end of each chapter in *Tappan's Handbook of Healing Massage Techniques* as homework or for in-class presentations. This offers learning opportunities beyond simple recall.

*The lecture outlines and test bank are available in the printed Instructor's Resource Manual and on CD-ROM using PowerPoint® software.

EVALUATION OF KNOWLEDGE AND SKILLS

- Use the test bank in the *Instructor's Resource Manual* to create written exams.*

- Fill-in-the-blank questions from the end of the chapter study guides in *Tappan's Handbook of Healing Massage Techniques* can be added to written exams.

- Video segment questions from the CD-ROM and in the *Instructor's Resource Manual* can be added to written exams.

- Use the performance evaluation forms in Appendix D of *Tappan's Handbook of Healing Massage Techniques* for practical testing.

*The lecture outlines and test bank are available in the printed Instructor's Resource Manual and on CD-ROM using PowerPoint® software.

SYLLABUS

COURSE: Massage Therapy Theory

TEXTBOOK: Benjamin, P. and Tappan, F. *Tappan's Handbook of Healing Massage Techniques,* 4th edition, Prentice Hall, Upper Saddle River, 2005.

OBJECTIVES: On completion of this course, you will have foundation knowledge for understanding and applying massage therapy. You will gain insight into the philosophical and historical background of massage therapy, the effects and clinical applications of massage, and contraindications and endangerment sites. You will learn general guidelines for giving massage including the therapeutic relationship and ethics, setting up the physical environment, and elements of performance.

CONTENTS:

Unit 1   Healing Massage—A Wellness Perspective

Unit 2   History of Massage

Unit 3   Effects and Benefits of Massage

Unit 4   Clinical Applications of Massage

Unit 5   Endangerment Sites, Contraindications, Cautions

Unit 6   Guidelines for Giving Massage—The Therapeutic Relationship

Unit 7   Guidelines for Giving Massage—Practical Considerations

REQUIREMENTS:

1. Complete reading assignments.
2. Give presentation on selected topic.

EVALUATION

1. Presentation will count as $\frac{1}{4}$ of the grade.
2. Unit quizzes will count as $\frac{1}{4}$ of the grade.
3. Final examination will count as $\frac{2}{4}$ of the grade.

Course: Massage Therapy Theory

Sample Weekly Schedule

15 week semester; 3 hours per week = 45 hours

Week	Unit	Topic
1	1	Healing massage—a wellness perspective
2	2	Early history of massage
3		Modern history of massage
4	3	Effects of massage tissue and organ systems level
5		Effects of massage organ systems and organism level
		Holistic view of effects
6	4	Clinical applications of massage
7		Clinical applications of massage (cont.)
8	5	Endangerment sites, contraindications, cautions
9		Contraindications and cautions (cont.)
10	6	Therapeutic relationship and ethics
11		Therapeutic relationship and ethics (cont.)
12	7	Equipment, positioning and draping, self-care
13		Performance elements, presentations
14	—	Presentations, course review
15	—	Final examination

SYLLABUS

COURSE: Western Massage

TEXTBOOK: Benjamin, P. and Tappan, F. *Tappan's Handbook of Healing Massage Techniques*, 4th Edition, Prentice Hall, Upper Saddle River, N.J., 2005.

OBJECTIVES: On completion of this course, you will have knowledge and skills to perform Western massage techniques, joint movements, a full-body Western massage, and regional applications. You will learn to perform variations of techniques in the seven basic Western massage technique categories, how to combine techniques into full-body sessions, and how to apply techniques in therapeutic approaches to different body regions. The uses of hydrotherapy and thermal therapies with massage will be covered.

CONTENTS:

Unit 1   Western Massage Techniques

Unit 2   Joint Movements

Unit 3   Full-Body Western Massage

Unit 4   Applications for the Head and Face, Neck

Unit 5   Applications for the Back

Unit 6   Applications for the Lower Extremities and Buttocks

Unit 7   Applications for the Upper Extremities

Unit 8   Applications for the Chest and Abdomen

Unit 9   Hydrotherapy and Thermal Therapy

REQUIREMENTS:

1. Complete reading assignments.
2. Practice techniques and applications outside of class.

EVALUATION

1. Written examinations for Units 1, 2, 3, 4–9
2. Performance evaluation of Western massage techniques
3. Performance evaluation of joint movements
4. Performance evaluation of full-body Western massage
5. Performance evaluation of regional applications

Sample Weekly Schedule (150 hours course length; 2 semesters)

15 week semester; 5 hours per week = 75 hours

Semester I

Week	Unit	Topic
1	1	Introduction to Western massage; table set-up; overview of seven technique categories, review of draping and body mechanics; demonstration and practice on the back: applying oil, basic effleurage, kneading of shoulders
2		Overview of effleurage; demonstration and practice of effleurage variations on different body regions; review of performance elements
3		Overview of petrissage; demonstration and practice of petrissage variations; practice sequence combining effleurage and petrissage
4		Overview of friction; demonstration and practice of friction variations; practice sequence combining effleurage, petrissage, and friction
5		Review of endangerment sites, contraindications and cautions; overview of tapotement; demonstration and practice of tapotement variations; practice sequence combining effleurage, petrissage, and tapotement
6		Overview of vibration; demonstration and practice of vibration variations; use of electric vibrators, practice sequence combining techniques learned
7		Overview of touch without movement; demonstration and practice of touch without movement; practice sequence combining techniques learned
8		Written examination for Unit 1; performance evaluation of Western massage techniques (see Appendix D in *Tappan's Handbook of Healing Massage Techniques*)
9	2	Introduction to joint movements; general principles of joint movements; contraindications and cautions; overview of the neck region; mobilizing and stretching techniques for the neck; practice sequence combining massage and joint movements for the neck
10		Overview of the shoulder girdle area; mobilizing and stretching techniques for the shoulder; practice sequence combining massage and joint movements for the shoulder
11		Overview of the upper extremities; mobilizing and stretching techniques for the elbow, wrist, and hand; practice sequence combining massage and joint movements for the upper extremities
12		Overview of the chest area; mobilizing and stretching techniques for the rib cage and muscles that attach in the region; practice sequence combining massage and joint movements for the chest
13		Overview of the buttocks and lower extremities; mobilizing and stretching techniques for the hips, knees, ankles, and feet; practice sequence combining massage and joint movements for the lower extremities
14		Review of joint movements; practice of massage and joint movement routines
15		Written examination for Unit 2; performance evaluation of joint movements (See Appendix D in *Tappan's Handbook of Healing Massage Techniques*)

Semester II

Week	Unit	Topic
1	3	Introduction to full-body Western massage; general guidelines; demonstration of a full-body routine with discussion; practice sequence to review positioning, draping, body mechanics, and basic techniques
2		Practice massage routine with client prone
3		Practice massage routine with client prone (cont.)
4		Practice massage routine with client supine
		Practice massage routine with client supine
5		Practice massage routine with client in side-lying position
6		Full-body massage routine
7		Written examination for Unit 3; performance evaluation for full-body massage routine (see Appendix D in *Tappan's Handbook of Healing Massage Techniques*)
8	4	Introduction to regional applications of massage; overview of the neck, head, and face; therapeutic progression for the neck, head, and face; practice of neck, head, and face massage
9	5	Overview of the back; therapeutic progression for the back; practice of back massage
10	6	Overview of the buttocks region; therapeutic progression for the buttocks; overview of the lower extremities; foot massage routine; routine for enhancing mobility in the lower extremities
11	7	Overview of the upper extremities; routine for enhancing mobility in the upper extremities; routine for preventing forearm strain
12	8	Overview of chest and abdomen; massage routine to address rounded shoulders; massage routine for enhancing respiration
13	9	Thermal therapies; review of regional applications of massage
14		Integrating regional applications into full-body massage
15		Written examination for Units 4–9; performance evaluation of regional applications (see Appendix D in *Tappan's Handbook of Healing massage Techniques*)

SYLLABUS

COURSE: Hydrotherapy

TEXTBOOK: Benjamin, P. and Tappan, F. *Tappan's Handbook of Healing Massage Techniques*, 4th Edition, Prentice Hall, Upper Saddle River, N.J., 2005.

OBJECTIVES: On completion of this course, you will have basic knowledge of hydrotherapy and thermal therapies and their use in conjunction with massage. You will review the history of hydrotherapy as a natural healing art. The effects of different forms of hydrotherapy and thermal therapies will be presented, as well as general guidelines, cautions, and contraindications. Their applications before, after, and in conjunction with massage will be discussed.

CONTENTS:
Unit 1   History of Hydrotherapy
Unit 2   Hydrotherapy in Spas and Health Clubs
Unit 3   Thermal Therapy—Hot Applications
Unit 4   Thermal Therapy—Cold Applications

REQUIREMENTS:

1. Complete reading assignments.
2. Case study including written report and presentation on the use of hydrotherapy or thermal therapy in conjunction with massage in one of the following settings: spa, health club, physical therapy clinic, or athletic training room.

EVALUATION

1. Case study written report and presentation will count as $\frac{1}{4}$ of the grade.
2. Performance evaluation will count as $\frac{1}{4}$ of the grade.
3. Written examination will count as $\frac{1}{2}$ of the grade.

Course: Hydrotherapy

Sample Weekly Schedule

3-hour class period × 10 classes = 30 hours
or
5-hour class period × 10 classes = 50 hours

Week	Unit	Topic
1	1	History of hydrotherapy as a natural healing art and science
2	2	Healing properties of water, temperature ranges for hydrotherapy and thermal therapy, effects of thermo- and cryohydrotherapy
3		Hydrotherapy facilities in spas and health clubs: whirlpool bath, showers, steam rooms, steam cabinet, sauna, facial steam
4		Spa and health club facilities: field trip
5	3	Thermal therapy: hot applications demonstration
6	4	Thermal therapy and first aid: cold applications demonstration
7		Thermal therapy: massage applications practice
8		Physical therapy clinic or athletic training room: field trip
9		Case study presentations, performance evaluation
10		Case study presentations (cont.), written examination

SYLLABUS

COURSE: Asian Bodywork Therapy—Theory

TEXTBOOK: Benjamin, P. and Tappan, F. *Tappan's Handbook of Healing Massage Techniques,* 4th Edition, Prentice Hall, Upper Saddle River, NJ, 2005.

OBJECTIVES: On completion of this course, you will have foundation knowledge for understanding and applying Asian bodywork therapies (ABT) based on traditional Asian medicine, including Chinese meridian and acupoint theory. You will gain insight into the philosophical and historical background of Asian bodywork therapy and the essential differences between Western and traditional Asian medicine. You will also learn the principles of good body mechanics for applying ABT pressure techniques.

CONTENTS:

Unit 1   History of Asian Bodywork Therapy
Unit 2   Basic Concepts of Traditional Asian Medicine
Unit 3   Energy Channels and the Chinese Body Clock
Unit 4   Acupoints
Unit 5   Application of ABT Pressure Techniques

REQUIREMENTS:

1. Complete reading assignments.
2. Give presentation on a selected topic (e.g., a specific form of ABT).

EVALUATION:

1. Presentation will count as $\frac{1}{4}$ of the grade.
2. Two quizzes will count as $\frac{1}{8}$ of the grade.
3. Performance evaluation of ABT pressure techniques will count as $\frac{1}{8}$ of the grade.
4. Final examination will count as $\frac{2}{4}$ of the grade.

Sample Weekly Schedule

15 week semester for 3 hours per week = 45 hours

Week	Unit	Topic
1	1	History of traditional Asian medicine
2	2	Basic concepts of traditional Asian medicine
3		Basic concepts of traditional Asian medicine (cont.)
4		Basic concepts of traditional Asian medicine (cont.)
5	3	Energy channels and Chinese body clock
6		Energy channels and Chinese body clock (cont.)
7		Energy channels and Chinese body clock (cont.)
8	4	Acupoints
9		Acupoints (cont.)
10		Acupoints (cont.)
11	5	Application of ABT pressure techniques
12		Application of ABT pressure techniques (cont.)
13		Student presentations
14		Student presentations and final written exam
15		Performance evaluation

1

Healing Massage— A Wellness Perspective

LECTURE OUTLINE

I. Massage as a Natural Healing Art
   A. Natural healing arts
      1. Healing gifts of nature
      2. Massage as manual therapy
   B. Natural healing philosophy
      1. Origins in nineteenth century (also see Chapter 2)
      2. Preference for natural healing methods
      3. Innate healing force
      4. Holistic view of human life
   C. The nature of healing
      1. To make healthy, whole, or sound
      2. A force from within, recipient an active participant
      3. Contrast to *curing*, an outside force, recipient a passive participant
   D. Holistic
      1. The wholeness of human beings
      2. Body, mind, emotions, spirit

II. Definition of Massage
   A. Massage defined
      1. Intentional and systematic soft tissue manipulation
      2. Joint movements and stretching included
      3. Primary characteristics are *touch* and *movement*
   B. Massage technique described as action and intention
      1. Actions such as sliding, kneading, rubbing
      2. Intention is the aim that guides the action
         a. Determines choice of technique
         b. Guides the action in subtle ways
   C. Massage and bodywork as a general category

III. Massage and Bodywork Traditions *[See Figure 1-1 Map of World Traditions of Massage and Bodywork]*
   A. Four world traditions of massage

B. Folk and native massage traditions *[Also see Chapter 2]*
   1. Specific to a group of people defined by location
   2. Passed down through apprenticeship from elders
   3. Based on past practices and experience
   4. Larger context includes herbal remedies, rituals, religious beliefs
C. Ayurvedic massage tradition *[Also see Chapter 2]*
   1. Originated in India in about 500 B.C.E.
   2. Ancient text called the Vedas
   3. Massage helps circulate *vayu* or wind in *siras* or vessels
   4. Balances energy in *charkas*
   5. Oils chosen carefully for the individual
D. Asian bodywork therapy tradition *[Also see Chapters 2, 17–20]*
   1. Roots in traditional Chinese medicine
   2. Based on energy channels and acupoints
E. Western massage tradition *[Also see Chapters 7–11]*
   1. Seven Western massage technique categories *[See Figure 1-2 Seven Basic Western Massage Technique Categories; CD-ROM Video]*
      a. Effleurage
      b. Petrissage
      c. Friction
      d. Tapotement
      e. Vibration
      f. Touch without movement
      g. Joint movements
   2. Contemporary massage and bodywork is based primarily on Western science (e.g., myofascial massage, trigger point therapy, lymphatic drainage massage)
   3. The eclectic practitioner combines and synthesizes different approaches

IV. Massage and Western Medicine *[Also see Chapter 2]*
  A. Massage as alternative therapy (either/or)
  B. Massage as complementary therapy (secondary to primary treatment)
  C. Complementary and alternative medicine (CAM) (broad range of therapies)
  D. Integrative health care (many options for healing an individual)

V. Wellness Perspective
  A. The concept of wellness
   1. Beyond the old idea of health as the absence of disease
   2. Goal of achieving a vibrant meaningful life
  B. Travis's Illness/Wellness Continuum *[See Figure 1-3 The Illness/Wellness Continuum]*
   1. Wellness model
   2. Treatment model
   3. High-level wellness *[See Table 1-1 Components of Wellness and a Healthy Lifestyle]*
  C. Wellness Massage Pyramid (WMP) *[See Figure 1-4 Wellness Massage Pyramid]*
   1. Seven levels of the WMP
      a. Treatment for illness or injury
      b. Recovery from illness or injury
      c. Prevention of illness or injury
      d. Neutral zone
      e. Health maintenance
      f. Personal growth
      g. Enjoyment of life

2. WMP as a tool
    a. To explain reasons people seek massage
    b. To describe the goals of a massage session

VI. Wellness and the Health Professions
    A. Massage in the scope of several health professions
    B. Massage therapists work in the full range of the Wellness Pyramid
    C. Physical therapists and nurses working in health care concentrate on the foundation levels of the Wellness Pyramid in treatment, recovery, prevention

VII. Terminology
    A. Options
        1. Clients, guests, patients, recipient of massage
        2. Practitioners, massage therapists, therapists, giver of massage
        3. Sessions, treatments, procedures
    B. Distinguishing between wellness and treatment terminology *[See Table 1–2 Wellness/ Treatment Terminology Chart]*

SUGGESTED CLASSROOM ACTIVITIES

- Invite a panel of three to five massage practitioners from a variety of settings (health club, spa, hospital, nursing home, chiropractic, or private practice) to discuss their approaches to massage and to answer student questions. Variation: Invite a single presenter from a setting especially relevant to the students.

- Invite a panel of three to five massage practitioners from different massage traditions, approaches, or forms to discuss their approaches to massage and to answer student questions. Variations: Invite a single presenter who practices a form of massage especially relevant to the students.

- Arrange for demonstrations of massage from different traditions, or different forms of massage and bodywork. Conduct a class discussion about similarities and differences. Variation: Show videos of different forms of massage and bodywork.

- Have students interview people who have received massage in the past year, and ask why they sought massage in the first place and the benefits they think they received. Discuss in class using the Wellness Massage Pyramid.

- Assign reading of the White House Commission Report on CAM Policy (www.whccamp .hhs.com). Use as a basis of class discussion about the current and future acceptance of CAM therapies, including massage.

- Invite a presenter from an integrative health care setting to discuss his or her philosophy of healing and the place of massage therapy in that setting.

2

History of Massage

LECTURE OUTLINE

I. Massage as an ancient and global health and healing practice.
   A. Massage is found in every known culture in the world. *[Refer to Figure 1-1 Map of World Traditions of Massage and Bodywork]*
      1. The practice of massage has evolved as cultures come in contact with one another and ideas are exchanged.
      2. Massage therapy in North America is based on Western massage, but massage forms from other parts of the world are also having an influence.
      3. Knowledge of massage history can help practitioners appreciate the vast heritage of which they are a part.
      4. Massage from different time periods and places can be understood within the broad scope of the wellness perspective.
      5. Some forms of massage and bodywork are not only historical, having been developed long ago, but are also contemporary as they continue to be practiced today.
   B. Native and Folk Traditions
      1. Knowledge and skills handed down through apprenticeship and oral tradition have left little historical evidence.
      2. Two sources of historical information for folk and native traditions are
         1. Written reports of explorers who first came in contact with indigenous peoples.
         2. Old traditions of massage that continue to be practiced today.
      3. South Sea Islands
         a. Reports from European and American explorers in the South Sea Islands (Pacific Ocean) in the 1700–1800s.
         b. In New Zealand the Maoris practiced *romi-romi* and massage for clubfoot in infants.
         c. On Tonga Island *toogi-toogi* was performed to relieve fatigue and promote good sleep.
         d. In the Sandwich Islands (Hawaii) natives practice *lomi-lomi* to relieve soreness, fatigue, and promote sleep. *[Refer to quote by Nordhoff 1874 in Chapter 2, p. 21]*
      4. Curanderas
         a. Curanderas are traditional Hispanic healers found in the southwestern United States and Mexico.

      b. Elements of folk traditions of eighth-century Spain, and Aztecs of Mexico.

      c. Combines herbs, midwifery, ritual practices, and massage.

      d. *Sobardoras* are curanderas who specialize in massage, also using herbs and "boneset-ting" techniques.

C. Ancient Civilizations

  1. From Sumer in 2100 B.C.E., a clay tablet describes a remedy of herbs and "rubbing" and "frictions." *[Refer to quote from Time-Life Book 1987 in Chapter 2, p. 21]*

  2. China and Japan

      a. A form of seated bodywork given by "barbers" has been available in China for centuries. *[See Figure 2-1 Chinese Barber Performing a Form of Percussion on a Seated Patron in China in the 1790s]*

      b. The Yellow Emperor's Classic of Internal Medicine c. 500 B.C.E. describes essential elements of traditional Chinese medicine.

      c. Ancient Chinese healing techniques included acupuncture, acupressure, massage, and movements forms such as tai chi and qi gong.

      d. Amma is traditional Japanese massage brought from China via Korean peninsula in sixth century C.E.

      e. Shiatsu is modern form of Japanese massage derived from amma and Western science and developed by Torujiro Namikoshi in the 1940s.

[See Chapters 17–20 for more information about the history of Asian massage and bodywork]

  3. India

      a. The Vedas c. 500 B.C.E. describe Ayurveda or "knowledge of long life," ancient health practices of India.

      b. Ayurvedic health practices include vegetarian eating, cleansing, movements and postures (yoga), breathing exercises, meditation, and massage.

      c. Ayurveda popularized today by Deepak Chopra.

      d. Today's infant massage partly based on the ancient practice of massaging babies in India.

  4. Greece

      a. Hippocrates (450–377 B.C.E.) wrote of using "frictions" to treat sprains and dislocations, and recommended abdominal kneading and chest clapping.

      b. Aristotle (384–322 B.C.E.) recommended massage as a remedy for weariness.

      c. Alexander the Great (356–323 B.C.E.) had a personal massage specialist to "rub" him and prepare his bath.

      d. Massage was given in the ancient Greek gymnasium. *[Refer to description by Galen c. 130–200 C.E. in Chapter 2, p. 23]*

  5. Rome

      a. Celsus (25 B.C.E.–50 C.E.), a Roman physician wrote *De Medicina,* which described "frictions" and "unctions" as treatment methods.

      b. Roman baths offered exercise, hot and cold baths, and massage
[Refer to description of massage by Seneca (4 B.C.E.–65 C.E.) in Chapter 2, p. 24]

      c. Turkish baths developed from Roman baths.

         1. Popular in cities of Europe and United States in nineteenth century.

         2. Vigorous form of bodywork given at Turkish baths. *[Refer to quote in Johnson 1866 in Chapter 2]*

         3. Modern health club retains elements of Roman and Turkish baths offering exercise, swimming, showers, steam room, sauna, whirlpool, and massage.

D. Middle Ages and Renaissance Europe

  1. Middle Ages extended from sixth to fourteenth centuries in Europe.

      a. Classical writings of Greeks and Romans were lost in Europe but were preserved by Arabic people in the Near East and by Irish monks.

      b. Use of "frictions" and "rubbing" was preserved in folk traditions of Europe.

      c. Book called *Tacuinum Sanitatis* in Latin c. 1000 describes a holistic view of health and disease.

      d. Avicenna (980–1137 C.E.) an Arabic physician, wrote about massage in a medical text. *[See quote from Wood and Becker 1981 in Chapter 2, p. 25]*

  2. Renaissance is dated approximately fourteenth to seventeenth centuries in Europe.

      a. Classical writings of Greeks and Romans were reintroduced into Europe, and interest in massage as treatment was revived.

      b. Ambrose Pare (1517–1590) wrote about "frictions" for joint stiffness and wound healing.

II. Western Massage—Nineteenth and Early Twentieth Centuries

  A. Pehr Henrick Ling (1776–1839)

    1. Fencing master, poet, playwright, educator, healer

    2. Developed four systems of movement or training: military, educational, aesthetic, and medical.

    3. Wrote *General Principles of Gymnastics,* published in 1840.

    4. Ling's system of Medical Gymnastics was known as the Swedish Movement Cure in United States. *[See Figure 2–2 Drawings from The Prevention and Cure of Many Chronic Diseases by Movements by Roth 1851]*

      a. Based on theory of "forces"

      b. Included active and passive movements

      c. Passive movements: shaking, hacking, pressing, stroking, pinching, squeezing, kneading, clapping, vibrations, rolling

      d. Treated diseases such as congestion, humming in the ears, gastritis, constipation, etc.

      e. Advocated study of anatomy and physiology with a holistic perspective *[Refer to quote by Ling 1840 in Chapter 2, p. 25]*

      f. Students from the Royal Institute of Gymnastics in Stockholm (est. 1813) took knowledge of Ling's work all over the world.

      g. Ling's legacy to massage practitioners includes a belief in the healing value of active and passive movements, holistic view of human beings, and the movements themselves.

  B. Johann Mezger (1838–1909)

    1. Physician in Amsterdam

    2. Divided soft tissue manipulation into four broad categories using French terms: effleurage, petrissage, tapotement, friction. *[See Figure 2–3 Drawings from Massage and the Original Swedish Movements by Ostrom 1905]*

    3. Mezger's work instrumental in reviving interest in massage in medical settings.

  C. Swedish Movement Cure in the United States

    1. Dr. Roth wrote first book in English on Ling's system in 1851, *Prevention and Cure of Many Chronic Diseases by Movements.*

    2. Swedish movement cure brought to United States by Dr. George Taylor of New York in 1854.

    3. Others who popularized Ling's work in the United States were Hartvig Nissen in Washington, D.C. (c. 1889), Baron Nils Posse in Boston (c. 1894), Kurre Ostrom in Philadelphia (c. 1905), Axel Grafsstrom in New York (c. 1904).

    4. By early twentieth century, Mezger's massage and the Swedish movement cure were being combined by practitioners and evolved into Swedish massage.

III. Western Massage—Early to Mid-Twentieth Century
   A. Massage in Conventional Medicine
      1. In 1700s called *frictions, rubbing, medical rubbing*
      2. Called the *anatriptic art* [**Refer to Johnson's book The Anatriptic Art, *1866*]**
      3. Lucas-Championniere (c. 1880) advocated soft tissue manipulation in treatment of bone fractures.
      4. Albert Hoffa published *Technik der Massage* in Germany in 1900.
      5. Douglas Graham published *A Treatise on Massage, Its History, Mode of Application and Effects* in 1902, which aroused interest in massage as a therapeutic agent in medical circles in United States.
      6. James B. Mennell (1880–1957)
         a. Lecturer at Training school of St. Thomas's Hospital in London from 1912 to 1935
         b. Wrote *Physical Treatment by Movement, Manipulation and Massage* in 1917
         b. Stressed care and gentleness in giving massage
         c. Influential in early physical therapy profession
      7. Reconstruction Aides
         a. Reconstruction Department created in U.S. Army in 1918
         b. Physiotherapy including massage was used to treat wounds of soldiers injured in World War I.
      8. C. M. Sampson described modalities used in the developing field of physical therapy in the textbook *A Practice of Physiotherapy* (1926) [**Refer to Figure 2–4 A Corner of the General Massage Section of an Army Hospital c. 1926**]
      9. Mary McMillan
         a. Pioneer in development of physical therapy in the United States
         b. Trained and worked in London hospitals
         c. Came to United States as director of Massage and Medical Gymnastics at Children's Hospital in Portland, Maine.
         d. Served as chief aide at Walter Reed Hospital and instructor of war emergency course for reconstruction aides during World War I.
         e. Wrote *Massage and Therapeutic Exercise* (1921) while Director of Physiotherapy at Harvard Medical School from 1921 to 1925.
      10. Physical therapists treated victims of the polio epidemic in the 1940s.
      11. Use of massage in physical therapy declined following World War II.
   B. Natural Health and Healing
      1. Philosophy of natural healing defined in the late nineteenth century
      2. J. Harvey Kellogg (1852–1943) advocated "biologic living," including massage, and was Director of the Battle Creek Sanitarium in Michigan.
      3. C. W. Post (1854–1914) opened a sanitarium (health resort) called La Vita Inn and taught relaxation techniques along with other natural health practices. [**Refer to quote by Post in Chapter 2, p. 29**]
      4. Bernarr MacFadden (1868–1955)
         a. Popularized natural health and healing.
         b. Opened a string of physical culture resorts in the East and Midwest United States in early 1900s.
         c. Published *Physical Culture Magazine*.
         d. Established MacFadden's Physical Culture Training School in Chicago and graduated doctors of "physcultopathy" based on the old Swedish movement cure.
      5. Swedish massage
         a. Heyday from 1920 to 1950

       b. Included massage, Swedish movements, hydrotherapy, heat lamps, diathermy, and colonic irrigation.

       c. College of Swedish Massage in Chicago trained practitioners of "scientific massage" in the 1930–1940s. *[See Figure 2–5 Women's Class in "Scientific Massage Techniques" c. 1940]*

       d. Graduates of Swedish massage training programs also worked in massage parlors, beauty parlors, health clubs, resorts, hospitals, and with professional sports teams, and with unconventional doctors such as chiropractors and naturopaths.

   C. Sports

      1. Sports massage can be traced to ancient Greek times (See "Ancient Greek Gymnasium" this chapter)

      2. The rubdown for athletes was well established in the United States and Europe by the late 1800s.

       a. Rubdown consisted of superficial skin friction with the hand, brush, coarse towel, or horsehair glove.

       b. H. Joseph Fay described vigorous kneading "to rid the muscles of waste" in *Scientific Massage for Athletes* in 1916.

       c. Harry Andrews described "rubbing, stroking, pinching, and slapping" to "arouse latent energy and reinvigorate the limbs" of athletes. *[See Figure 2–6 Harry Andrews, Trainer and Masseur, Massaging the Leg of an Athlete c. 1910]*

      3. Albert Baumgartner, former trainer at the State University of Iowa

       a. Wrote *Massage in Athletics* in 1947.

       b. Described massage as used in preparation for workout or competition, during rest periods between activities, for recuperation, and for minor injuries.

      4. By 1950s massage had largely disappeared from the sports scene.

      5. Sports massage was revived in the 1970s within the growing field of massage therapy.

   D. Fitness at the YMCA

      1. Tradition of massage at YMCA was established by early 1900s

      2. R. Tait McKenzie described workouts at the YMCA in 1915 as consisting of a mixture of Swedish gymnastics and games, followed by a bath and a rubdown.

      3. *[Refer to quote about general wellness massage offered at the YMCA in 1953 in Chapter 2, p. 32]*

IV. Later Twentieth Century United States

   A. Period of decline in the 1950s

   B. Esalen Massage in the 1970s

      1. Massage revived in 1960s as part of the Human Potential Movement and counterculture.

      2. Form of massage developed at the Esalen Institute in Big Sur, California

      3. Loosely based on Western massage emphasizing sensual aspects of massage *[Refer to quote from The Massage Book 1972 in Chapter 2]*

   C. 1970s were a period of opening to new ideas from other cultures and introduction of massage and bodywork from India and China into Western culture.

   D. Impact of the 1970s on massage and bodywork

      1. Significant growth in number of massage practitioners

      2. Increase in potential massage clients

      3. Number of training programs in massage therapy increased

      4. Concept of holistic health and healing revived

      5. Values of caring, heart, and connection became defining qualities of the work.

   E. Wellness Movement in 1970s

      1. Within fields of health, physical education, recreation

2. John Travis, M.D. [*See Figure 1-3 Illness/Wellness Continuum,* **and** *Figure 1-4 Components of Wellness and a Healthy Lifestyle*]
3. Idea of wellness programs spread to medical settings, for example, hospital programs that teach good health habits and illness prevention.
F. National Association of Nurse Massage Therapists established in 1987.

V. Milestones at the Turn of the Twenty-First Century
A. Increase in research about massage therapy
B. AMTA Foundation, an American Massage Therapy Association affiliate, incorporated in 1992 and research database made available on its Web site in 2001.
C. Touch Research Institute at the University of Miami founded in 1992
D. Office of Alternative Medicine
1. Established at National Institutes of Health (NIH) in 1992
2. Elevated to National Center of Complementary and Alternative Medicine in 1998
E. National Certification Examination for Therapeutic Massage and Bodywork first given in 1992
F. "Unconventional Medicine in the United States" appeared in the *New England Journal of Medicine* in 1993, confirming growth in use of CAM therapies by consumers.
G. First International Symposium on the Science of Touch held in May 2002
H. White House Commission on Complementary and Alternative Medicine Final Report made in 2002.
I. Commission on Massage Therapy Accreditation (COMTA) received United States Department of Education (USDE) approval in 2002.
J. American Massage Therapy Association (AMTA) opinion survey reports increasing acceptance and use of massage by consumers of all ages (2002).

SUGGESTED CLASSROOM ACTIVITIES

- Take a field trip to a historic site such as a Turkish bath, hot springs, YMCA, resort, or other place where massage has been available for decades. Get a tour of the facilities from someone knowledgeable about its history.

- Invite in a speaker who learned massage in the 1970s or earlier time period. Have him or her talk about what their initial training was like and how the use of massage has changed in the field over the past 30 or more years.

- Have students portray massage practitioners from different time periods and cultures that interest them. Presentations could take the form of role playing, with the student describing their character's training, type of massage, and other information that puts their work in historical context.

- Show movie clips of massage from films set in historical time periods. Discuss the type of massage given and how historically accurate the depictions of massage seem. Examples: *Ben Hur* (baths in ancient Rome); *Chariots of Fire* (trainer and masseur in nineteenth century); *Pat and Mike* (trainer and masseur in 1950s); *Shower* (Chinese bath house massage in twentieth century).

- Have students "show and tell" about a historical object (e.g., old vibrator or oil bottle), book, newspaper or magazine article, or advertisement they found through research in a library, old book or antique store.

- Develop a collection of objects, books, articles, advertisements, and so on related to the history of massage that can be used for student assignments or as visual aids for teaching.

3

Effects and Benefits of Massage

LECTURE OUTLINE

I. Effects of Massage *[See Table 3–1 Summary of the Effects of Massage on the Body-Mind]*
   A. The effects of massage are changes in the body, mind, and emotions of the recipient during a massage session.
   B. Examples of effects: muscles relaxation, increased alertness, reduced anxiety
   C. Different massage techniques produce different effects
   D. Practitioners who can apply techniques to produce specific effects will be more successful in achieving session or treatment goals.

II. Tissue Level
   A. Massage improves overall health of tissues primarily by increasing blood and lymph circulation
   B. Tissue repair
      1. Massage is contraindicated in the immediate location of the injury during the *inflammatory phase*, especially with infection.
      2. In the *regeneration phase*, circulatory massage facilitates removal of damaged cells, excess fluid, and byproducts of inflammation; and transports building blocks for new tissue formation.
      3. In the *remodeling phase*, deep transverse or Cyriax friction can help in formation of healthy scar tissue.
      4. Stress reduction massage helps the body heal wounds faster.
   C. Connective Tissue (CT)
      1. Three classifications of connective tissue
         a. Fluid (e.g., blood and lymph)
         b. Supporting (e.g., cartilage and bone)
         c. CT proper (ligaments, tendons, fascia)
      2. Thixotropy
         a. Characteristic of CT so that it becomes more fluid and pliable when mobile, and firmer when less mobile.
         b. Massage techniques that involve pressing, friction, stretching, and other movements raise the temperature and energy level of connective tissue making it be more pliable.

3. Prevention of CT abnormalities and dysfunction (e.g., kneading and deep friction can help prevent a condition called *fibrosis*)
4. Fascia
    a. Adhesions in fascia can be "unstuck" with massage techniques such as kneading, skin rolling, deep transverse friction, broadening techniques, and myofascial massage. *[Refer to Chapter 12 Myofascial Massage]*

III. Organ System Level
  A. Integumentary System
    1. Review components of integumentary system
    2. Massage stimulates sensory receptors for
        a. General relaxation
        b. Body awareness
        c. Pain reduction
        d. Promotes healthy infant development
    3. Massage unblocks skin pores through
        a. Frictions and rubbing of the skin
        b. Bathing and hydrotherapy
        c. Scraping or friction with towel or tool
    4. Massage promotes skin moisture by
        a. Increased perspiration
        b. Increased activity of sebaceous glands
        c. Addition of oil or lotion
    5. Massage promotes formation of healthy scar tissue
        a. Use cross-fiber and with fiber techniques
        b. May also reduce scar thickness
  B. Skeletal System
    1. Review of components of skeletal system
    2. General bone and joint health promoted by good circulation
    3. Healthy, pliable, relaxed muscles and connective tissue surrounding joints allow optimal range of motion and alignment.
    4. Flexibility at joints enhanced with massage and stretches
    5. Joint movements stimulate production of synovial fluid
  C. Muscular System
    1. Review of components of muscular system
    2. Importance of muscular system for overall health
    3. Many aches and pains caused by problems in the musculature
    4. Cellular level
        a. Muscles maintain normal cellular level activity and balance through movement.
        b. *Underactivity* leads to poor circulation, accumulation of waste products, poor cellular nutrition
        c. *Overactivity* leads to insufficient nutrients and oxygen, accumulation of waste products, muscle tension.
        d. Massage mimics muscle contraction helping to minimize effects of under- and overactivity
    5. Massage helps *hypertonic* muscles return to a relaxed state through
        a. Reduction of general muscle tension through activation of parasympathetic nervous system (relaxation response)
        b. Conscious letting go of tension with passive state during massage session

    c. Increased sensory stimulation leading to normalization of muscle tone as reflex pathways rebalance themselves

    d. Technique called *muscle approximation* reduces tone in specific muscle; works through muscle spindles

    e. *Origin and insertion technique* uses cross-fiber friction to muscle attachments to reduce overall muscle tone; works through Golgi tendon organs.

6. Increased joint mobility and flexibility

    a. Flexibility is a function of the combined muscular, skeletal, and nervous systems

    b. Factors that can restrict movement at joints

       1. Hypertonic muscles

       2. Scarring in muscle and connective tissue

       3. Myofascial adhesions

       4. Trigger points *[Refer to Chapter 13 Neuromuscular Therapy]*

       5. General connective tissue thickening and rigidity

    c. Massage and joint movements help maintain joint mobility and flexibility by addressing any abnormal conditions in soft tissues surrounding joints

    d. A study found that massage increased range of motion in hamstrings using effleurage, stretching effleurage, kneading and deep friction.

7. Posture

    a. Proper body alignment is combined function of the muscular, skeletal, and nervous systems. Review good posture.

    b. Poor posture results from a combination of factors such as

       1. Ergonomically inadequate workstations and tools

       2. Injuries

       3. Poor postural habits

    c. Poor posture leads to

       1. Imbalances between muscle groups

       2. Hypertonic and shortened muscles

       3. Fascial adhesions

       4. Trigger points

       5. Other problem conditions

    d. Vice versa, muscle imbalances or pathologies may result in poor body alignment

    e. Strategies used in massage therapy to address body alignment:

       1. Analyze client's posture and identifying probable factors in misalignment

       2. Apply massage and related movements with goal of proper alignment (e.g., relaxing and elongating muscles, lengthening muscle groups with stretching, breaking fascial adhesions with myofascial techniques, relieving trigger points).

D. Nervous and Endocrine Systems

  1. Review of nervous and endocrine systems structures and function

  2. Effects of massage related to the nervous system include

    a. Stimulation of sensory receptors helps sharpen body awareness

    b. Nervous system plays role in muscle relaxation and pain reduction

    c. Promotes proper development in infants through nervous system stimulation

  3. Some massage and joint movement techniques use the nervous system to effect desired results:

    a. Activate proprioceptors in muscles for relaxation and elongation

    b. Stimulate parasympathetic system for relaxation response

E. Cardiovascular System

  1. Review of cardiovascular system anatomy and function

  2. Benefits of increased circulation through massage

      a. Improved nutrient and oxygen delivery

      b. Clearance of metabolic wastes

      c. During tissue repair, transport of new building materials into the area, and removal of damaged cells

      d. Delivery of macrophages to attack body invaders

  3. Massage and increased blood circulation

      a. Studies show capillary vessel dilation and increased blood flow to areas receiving massage.

      b. Even using light pressure can help increase local blood flow.

      c. Superficial friction produces hyperemia in skin and underlying connective tissue; red and warm skin surface.

      d. Deep effleurage and petrissage increase blood flow that lasts for some time after the application.

  4. Venous return

      a. Mechanical action of deep effleurage enhances venous flow in limbs.

      b. Deep stroking on limbs should always be toward the heart (i.e., distal to proximal); prevents damage to valves in veins.

      c. Varicose veins

          1. Characterized by damaged values and pooled blood

          2. Blood clots can form in pooled blood

          3. Massage locally contraindicated over varicose veins

          4. Massage generally contraindicated with history of blood clots unless physician approval

      d. Mechanical action of effleurage and petrissage mimics muscle contraction and assists venous return.

      e. Venostasis is condition in which normal blood flow in veins is slowed or halted.

          1. May occur with inactivity, varicose veins, or edema of surrounding tissues

          2. Massage proximally first to open circulatory pathways

  5. Blood pressure

      a. Study shows that blood pressure is temporarily decreased for about 40 minutes after massage.

      b. Relaxation response decreases blood pressure, and saves wear and tear on circulatory system.

  6. Red blood cells (RBCs)

      a. Massage increases the number of circulating red blood cells, thereby increasing oxygen carrying capacity of the blood.

          1. RBCs stored in liver released during massage

          2. RBCs in stagnant capillary beds returned to circulation

F. Lymphatic System and Immunity

  1. Review of lymphatic system, fluid, and functions including immunity

  2. Lymph fluid movement

      a. Lymph is a viscous fluid

      b. Movement of fluid through lymph vessels largely dependent on outside forces

          1. Muscle contractions

          2. Action of diaphragm

          3. Pressure from tissues surrounding lymph capillaries

      c. Lack of movement leads to poor lymph circulation.

      d. Massage techniques such as effleurage and petrissage assist lymph flow mechanically.

      e. Special lymphatic massage techniques maximize lymph fluid entry into lymphatic capillaries. [Refer to Chapter 15 Lymphatic Drainage Massage]

3. Immunity
   a. Defined as "resistance to injuries and disease caused by specific foreign chemical compounds and pathogens."
   b. Massage enhances the immune response by improving lymph fluid flow and transport of lymphocytes.
   c. Massage is associated with improved immune function
      1. Activation of natural killer (NK) cells
      2. Decrease in cortisol levels
      3. Decrease in anxiety

G. Respiratory System
   1. Review of respiratory system structure and function
   2. Massage enhances respiratory function by
      a. Improving general blood circulation
      b. Encouraging relaxed diaphragmatic breathing
      c. Reducing tension and shortening in skeletal muscles involved in breathing
      d. Facilitating structural alignment and rib cage expansion for optimal vital capacity

H. Digestive System
   1. Review of digestive system structure and function
   2. Massage can improve digestion through
      a. Inducing parasympathetic nervous system activity
      b. Facilitating bowel movement thru abdominal massage
      c. Assisting bowel and gas movement in infants

I. Reproductive System
   1. Reproductive organs are not appropriate targets for therapeutic massage.
   2. The reproductive organs benefit from improved circulatory health as do all body systems.
   3. Massage as part of a stress reduction plan can contribute to improved sexual function.
   4. Massage for pregnant women
      a. Some massage practitioners work with midwives and other health professionals during delivery.
      b. Special application of Western massage, Asian bodywork therapy, and folk healing traditions
         1. During pregnancy to relieve discomforts
         2. During delivery to assist the process
   5. Breast massage
      a. Specialized skill
      b. Promotes function of lymphatic vessels and mammary glands
      c. Complementary therapy for women undergoing breast cancer treatment
      d. Requires informed consent
      e. May be beyond the legal scope of practice for some practitioners
   6. Penis erection
      a. May not indicate sexual arousal
         1. Result of increased blood flow to the area
         2. Erection will subside naturally if no arousal
      b. If result of sexual arousal, stop session immediately, inform client that session is over, leave the room, and discuss with client outside of immediate massage environment. Restate nonsexual nature of therapeutic massage.

IV. Organism Level
   A. Beyond the effects on one or two organ systems

B. Growth and development of infants
   1. Adequate pleasurable tactile experience in early life can influence desired traits such as calmness, gentleness, nonaggressiveness.
   2. Stimulation of tactile nerve endings in the skin helps the brain organize its circuitry for proper development.
   3. Movement and simulation of the kinesthetic sense also promote central nervous system development.
   4. Massage is an excellent way to provide systematic and regular touch and movement to growing infants.
C. Pain reduction
   1. Sensation of discomfort, distress, or suffering due to irritation or stimulation of sensory nerves and pain sensors.
   2. Muscle relaxation and improved local circulation can help relieve pain associated with tense muscles and accompanying lack of blood supply.
   3. Massage can be used to interrupt the pain-spasm-pain cycle caused by hypertonic muscles.
   4. Massage activates the neural-gating mechanism in the spinal cord through increased sensory stimulation.
      a. Larger, faster nerve fibers that carry sensory information block smaller, slower pain-transmitting nerve fibers.
      b. May be the source of temporary analgesia associated with deep transverse friction.
   5. Myofascial trigger points may be relieved with ischemic compression, stripping, and stretching techniques to the affected area.
   6. Massage induces release of endorphins and enkephalins—the body's natural pain killers.
D. Stress reduction
   1. Relaxation massage stimulates parasympathetic nervous system and the relaxation response.
      a. Decreased oxygen consumption and metabolic rate
      b. Increased intensity and frequency of alpha brain waves
      c. Reduced blood lactates
      d. Decreased blood pressure
      e. Reduced heart rate
      f. Slower respiration
      g. Decreased muscle tension
      h. Increased blood flow to internal organs
      i. Decreased anxiety, fear, phobia
      j. Increased positive mental health
      k. Improved quality of sleep
   2. Relaxation massage
      a. Application of effleurage and petrissage techniques
      b. Avoidance of specific techniques that cause discomfort
      c. Qualities such as light, smooth, flowing
      d. Enhanced with relaxing music, soft lighting, warm temperatures, and minimum talking
      e. Especially effective on the back
E. Mental and emotional effects
   1. Mental clarity
      a. Studies show that after receiving massage workers reported being more relaxed, in better moods, and more alert; students reported less anxiety and better memories.

      b. Job stress study found less fatigue, greater mental clarity, improved cognitive skills, and lower anxiety levels after regular 20-minute chair massage.
      c. Pre-event massage for athletes sparks stimulation and alertness for competition readiness.
      d. Massage for mental clarity is relatively short (8–20 minutes).
      e. Increased mental alertness could be related to
         1. Sensory stimulation
         2. Enhanced circulation to brain
         3. Calmer mind
  2. Emotional release
      a. Unexpressed emotions may come to the surface during massage.
      b. May take form of weeping, feelings of anger, fear or grief.
      c. May be due to relaxation and lowering of psychological defenses during massage
      d. May be important step in physical or psychological healing
      e. Mechanisms involved are little understood
  3. Feelings of general wellbeing may be the result of
      a. Relaxation response
      b. Release of endorphins
      c. Tactile pleasure
      d. Caring touch
      e. Reduction of pain and stress

V. Mechanisms of massage [See Table 3-2 Mechanisms to Explain the Effects of Massage]
  A. Theories about how massage works are based on
    1. Western biomedical model, anatomy and physiology
    2. Other theoretical systems such as Traditional Asian Medicine and Ayurvedic healing
    3. Cutting-edge mind-body studies
  B. Some effects of massage may be produced by more than one mechanism
  C. Specific massage techniques may produce a number of different effects
  D. Different sources of effects:
    1. Mechanical effects
      a. Result of physical forces such as compression, stretching, shearing, broadening, and vibration of body tissues
      b. Occur on gross level of physical structure
      c. Examples:
         1. Venous return using deep effleurage
         2. Elongation of muscles by stretching
         3. Increased lymph flow from kneading and deep effleurage
         4. Breaking tissue adhesions with shearing action of deep transverse friction
    2. Physiological effects
      a. Result of organic processes of the body at cellular, tissue, and organ system levels
      b. Examples:
         1. Relaxation response
         2. Anxiety reduction through release of endorphins
         3. Proper growth and development of infants from nervous system stimulation
    3. Reflex effects
      a. Functional change mediated by the nervous system
      b. Examples:
         1. Muscle relaxation
         2. Enhanced mental clarity

         3. Pain reduction via neural-gating mechanism
     c. Reflexology is type of bodywork in which reflex effects are thought to be involved, however, theories of how it works are not definitive.
  4. Body-mind effects
     a. Acknowledge the interplay of body, mind, emotions in health and disease
     b. Long tradition in healing systems all over the world
     c. New science of psychoneuroimmunology has grown from study of body-mind effects on health and disease
     d. Examples:
         1. Relaxation response
         2. Anxiety reduction
         3. Release of unexpressed emotions
  5. Energetic effects
     a. What energy is and how it relates to the body, health, and disease are yet to be determined in Western science.
     b. Ancient traditions of healing from China and India are based in part on theories of energy flow.
     c. Some forms of massage and bodywork aim to balance and improve the flow of energy.
     d. Many practitioners report feeling energy and its flow.
     e. Energy work is currently outside of understanding of Western science, however, it has persisted over time and is found to be useful by many people.
     f. Examples:
         1. Polarity therapy
         2. Therapeutic touch
         3. Reiki

VI. A Holistic View
  A. We live as whole persons and the effects of massage interact with each other in complex ways to produce an overall effect that is greater than the sum of its parts.
  B. The indivisible body and mind
    1. The body and mind function as a single unit (i.e., holistic).
    2. Physical manifestations of emotions include
      a. Blush of embarrassment
      b. Sweaty palms in nervousness
      c. Clenched fist of anger
      d. Wide-eyed fear
      e. Quickened heartbeat of love
    3. Body posture may reveal emotional states:
      a. Raised shoulders with fear
      b. Rounded shoulders with "weight of the world"
      c. Hunched shoulders for self-protection
    4. Connectedness of mind and body traced to our beginnings as embryos.
      a. Physical structures related to sensations are from the same embryonic source as those related to emotions.
      b. In touching the outermost part of the physical body, we are able to touch the innermost parts of our clients.
      c. Research on infant massage provides evidence for the connection of body and mind in humans.
  C. The *limbic system* is a group of structures within the brain associated with emotions and feelings.

1. Memory researchers have traced the relationship between touch memories and emotions.
2. Memories may be activated as well as created by touch.
3. Implications for massage practitioners
   D. *Character armor* is muscular tension caused by suppressed emotions.
   1. Examples of physical manifestations of suppressed emotions.
   2. In relaxing tense muscles, suppressed emotions may be felt.
   E. Massage has been called *body-centered therapy* since it works primarily through touch and movement of the body to enhance overall well-being.

VII. Benefits of Massage for Everyone
   A. When the effects of massage support general health and well-being or the ongoing healing process, there are *benefits* by definition.
   B. The main intention of wellness massage is to promote general and muscular relaxation and to enhance circulation of fluids, digestion, and elimination.
   C. Massage provides healthy touch which is a basic human need.

VII. Benefits for Special Populations *[Also see Chapter 4 Clinical Applications of Massage]*
   A. Examples of special populations that benefit from massage include pregnant women, infants, elderly, workers, athletes.
   B. Examples of those who benefit from psychological effects of massage include people in stressful life situations, in psychotherapy, with life-threatening illness, and in hospices.
   C. Even when treatment of a condition is not an option, massage may be used to improve the quality of life.

SUGGESTED CLASSROOM ACTIVITIES

- Analyze one or more research studies about the benefits of massage in more detail, noting the research question, subjects, methodology, results, and conclusions. Variation: Assign research studies to students for reporting to the class.

- Assign different body systems to students or student groups for class presentations on the system, effects of massage, and potential in treatment of pathologies related to the system.

- Demonstrate specific massage techniques that effect different body organs or systems.

- Demonstrate the connective tissue characteristic of thixotropy with a material such as clay, rubber bands, balloons, or any other material that becomes more pliable with movement.

- Analyze a student's alignment using a posture grid, and discuss how massage might be applied to help improve overall the body alignment. Variation: Pairs of students analyze each other's posture.

- Cut out pictures of people from old magazines and assign them to students as their clients. Show differences in age, gender, physical ability or disability, and other characteristics. Try to find pictures that show something about the client like their work, hobby, or sport activity. Have students work in groups to discuss their "client" and the ways they might benefit from massage given specific factors gleaned from the pictures. Present findings to the class. Variation: Students plan a massage session based on information from the pictures.

- Lead students through a deep breathing exercise. Have them describe from their experience what happens to their body and what muscles are involved. Discuss how massage might help in improving the ability to breathe deeply. (Refer to Chapter 10, Regional Applications of Massage, section on Massage for Respiration.)

- Put an anatomical model or chart that shows the internal organs on a massage table. Demonstrate how abdominal massage works mechanically to improve digestion and elimination, and why the direction of massage is clockwise. (Refer to Chapter 10, Regional Applications of Massage, section on Abdominal Massage.)

- Invite a pregnant woman to class to describe how her condition has affected her health and comfort. Discuss benefits of massage for her as an individual, plan a massage session for her as a class, and if there is time, demonstrate some techniques to address her needs. Variation: Invite an athlete, office worker, manual worker, elderly person.

- Invite a midwife who uses massage to describe its application during delivery.

- Lead students through a relaxation exercise (e.g., progressive relaxation) and have them observe their responses. Discuss in relation to the relaxation response and massage. Variation: Use a relaxation audiotape.

- When students seem to be getting drowsy and unfocused, lead them through a tapotement partner massage. This can be done in a "massage circle" while standing, or with the receiver sitting and the giver standing behind. Afterward, discuss the effect for improving mental clarity.

4

Clinical Applications of Massage

LECTURE OUTLINE

I. Clinical Massage Therapy
   A. Applications of massage for treatment of pathology
   B. Sources of information about clinical massage research

II. Value of Research
   A. Acceptance of massage in *integrated health care*
   B. *Evidence-based* means based on verifiable objective evidence (i.e., scientific research) *[Refer to quote on p. 67]*
   C. Applications of massage are more effective and safer with information from research.
   D. Aspects of massage can be measured objectively to provide valuable information
   E. Principle-based therapy
      1. In contrast to recipe- or formula-based *[Refer to quote on p. 68]*
      2. Treatment plan directed toward specific goals
      3. Considerations in session planning
         a. Condition being treated
         b. Tissue involvement
         c. Therapeutic potential of different treatment methods
         d. Patient centered rather than technique centered
   F. Research is most useful to add to understanding of effective applications of massage and not for developing treatment recipes
   G. *Research literacy*: understanding of scientific method, locating research articles, and reading, analyzing, and evaluating specific studies *[Refer to Table 4-1 Sources of Information about Clinical Applications of Massage]*

III. Clinical Approach
   A. Massage is *indicated* if it contributes to the alleviation of the diagnosed condition, or if it eases its symptoms.
   B. Massage is *contraindicated* if it would be detrimental to the client.
   C. *Client* in a clinical setting means "a person who is able to make choices about health care."
   D. Clinical benefits of massage therapy
      1. *Complementary* to a primary treatment method
      2. *Palliative care* to reduce symptoms and discomfort
      3. *Direct therapeutic effects* to help the body and mind heal
   E. Clinical massage therapy encompasses many different forms of massage.

IV. Musculo-Skeletal Pathologies
    A. Used in rehabilitation of injuries
    B. Direct therapeutic effects include
        1. Relieving muscle tension
        2. Increasing flexibility and range of motion
        3. Promoting healthy scar tissue
        4. Reducing muscular pain
    C. Pathologies and conditions treated with massage techniques
        1. Repetitive strain injuries (RSIs)
        2. Tension headache
        3. Low back pain
        4. Trigger points
        5. Fibromyalgia

V. Cardiovascular and Lymphatic Pathologies
    A. Relaxation massage for treating hypertension and cardiac arrhythmia
    B. Back massage for heart attack patients
    C. Therapeutic Touch reduced anxiety scores in patients in cardiovascular hospital unit.
    D. Edema and Lymphedema *[Refer to Chapter 14, Lymphatic Drainage Massage]*
        1. *Edema* is a condition of fluid buildup or swelling in tissues
            a. Occurs with muscular injuries, venostasis, prolonged standing
            b. Petrissage and effleurage applied distal to proximal helps reduce this type of edema
        2. *Lymphedema* is a specific type of edema caused by poor lymph circulation
            a. Example: After removal of lymph nodes during cancer surgery
            b. Permanent/regular treatment necessary for certain conditions
        3. Massage is contraindicated in cases of edema due to chronic cardiac, kidney, or liver problems
    E. Immune function
        1. Study of massage and HIV positive men—daily massage for a month
            a. Increase in number and activity of NK cells
            b. Reduced anxiety and stress
            c. Lower cortisol levels
            d. Increased serotonin levels
        2. Disease prevention measure for those with compromised immunity

VI. Respiratory Pathologies
    A. Benefits of massage for people with chronic bronchitis, emphysema, and asthma
        1. Anxiety reduction and relaxation that deepens breathing patterns
        2. Relaxation and lengthening of muscles tense from labored breathing *[Refer to Chapter 10, Regional Applications, section on Enhancing Respiration]*
        3. Reduced overall fatigue
        4. Loosen mucus for more productive coughs
            a. Passive movement of rib cage
            b. Percussion on the back and chest (refer to tapotement, cupping)
    B. Studies on children with asthma show positive results from massage.
        1. Lower anxiety
        2. Improved attitudes toward the asthma condition
        3. Increased peak airflow after regular massage by their parents
        4. Fewer asthma attacks over one-month period
        5. Daily massage may lead to improved airway tone, decreased airway irritability, better control of asthma in children

C. Study of Trager Psychophysical Integration®
   1. Trager bodywork consists of gentle, painless passive movements
   2. Received by patients with asthma, bronchitis, emphysema
   3. Movements applied to chest wall, neck, and abdomen
   4. Results included
      a. Improvement in vital capacity
      b. Improvement in respiratory rate
      c. Increased chest expansion
      d. Decreased anxiety and tension
D. Study of combination massage and neuromuscular (trigger point) therapy
   1. Received by chronic obstructive pulmonary disease (COPD) patients
   2. Techniques aimed at improving the function of chronically hypertonic muscles involved in breathing
   3. Results included
      a. Increase in thoracic gas volume
      b. Increase in peak flow and forced vital capacity
E. A variety of massage techniques can be used to achieve positive results
   1. Techniques effective at reducing stress
   2. Techniques effective for relaxing and freeing muscles of respiration
   3. Techniques effective for generally improving respiratory function

VII. Anxiety Reduciton in Hospitalized Patients
A. Value of massage for eliciting relaxation response and reducing anxiety
B. Studies of back massage by nurses
   1. Massage found to be effective, noninvasive technique for promoting relaxation and improving communication with institutionalized elderly
   2. Potential of massage for reducing dehumanizing effects of institutional care
C. Massage for hospitalized cancer patients
   1. Techniques: effleurage, petrissage, trigger point therapy
   2. Results included
      a. Reduced perceived level of pain and anxiety
      b. Increased feeling of relaxation
      c. Objective measures
         1. Decreased heart and respiratory rate
         2. Decreased blood pressure

VIII. Massage for Cancer Patients
A. Massage once listed as contraindication for cancer patients, now viewed as complementary therapy for cancer patients
B. General benefits of massage for cancer patients
   1. Reduced stress and anxiety
   2. Improved sleep
   3. Improved immune system function
   4. Pain relief
   5. Comfort of caring touch
C. Benefits for cancer surgery patients
   1. Faster recovery from anesthesia
   2. Faster wound healing
   3. Separation of adhesions around incisions
   4. Healthy scar formation
   5. Reduction of edema and lymphedema

6. Reduced pain and need for pain medication
7. Relief of soreness from prolonged bed rest
8. Improved circulation helps prevent pressure sores
D. Benefits for those in radiation and chemotherapy
    1. Reduces some negative side effects such as
        a. Fatigue
        b. Nausea
        c. Diarrhea
        d. Loss of appetite
        e. Insomnia
    2. Timing of massage related to receiving radiation or chemotherapy is an important consideration.
E. Benefits of massage on emotional level
    1. Relieves depression
    2. Offers pleasant social interaction to relieve isolation
    3. Reestablishes positive body image
    4. Empowers the patient to participate in their healing process
    5. Helps rebuild hope
F. Breast massage for post-mastectomy patients
G. Concerns about metastasis (i.e., spread of cancer)
    1. Always get doctors permission to massage cancer patient
    2. Avoid massage completely around site of tumor
    3. Avoid massage completely around site of recently removed tumor

IX. Pediatric Care
A. Touch Research Institute (TRI) at the University of Miami School of Medicine, Department of Pediatrics conducts research on massage for infants and children
B. Preterm infants benefit from tactile stimulation of massage
    1. Greater weight gain
    2. Increased motor activity
    3. More alert
    4. Improved performance on Brazelton Neonatal Behavioral Assessment Scale
    5. Techniques include
        a. Gentle stroking of head and neck, across the shoulders, from upper back to the waist, thighs to the feet, shoulders to hands
        b. Passive flexion/extension of arms and legs
C. Other pediatric applications
    1. Asthmatic children receiving 20-minute massage from mothers
       Results: decreased anxiety, improved moods of children and parents decreased cortisol levels, fewer attacks, better breathing
    2. Autistic children receiving one month of massage sessions
       Results: less touch sensitive, less distracted by sounds, more attentive in class, related more to teachers, better scores on Autism Behavior Checklist and Early Social Communications Scale
    3. Diabetic children given massage by their parents
       Results: lower anxiety, less depressed mood, insulin and food regulation scores improved, blood glucose levels decreased to normal range
    4. Depressed adolescent mothers given 10 massage session over 5 weeks
       Results: lower anxiety and stress, decrease in anxious behavior

5. Infants of depressed adolescent mothers given 15-minute massage, two times per week for six weeks
Results: gained more weight; improvement on emotional, social, and soothablity dimensions; improvement on face-to-face interaction ratings; less stress
6. Children with posttraumatic stress disorder massaged two times per week for a month
Results: less depression, lower anxiety, lower stress

X. Psychological Aspects of Treatment
  A. Massage reduces anxiety of hospitalized patients.
  B. Massage is complementary therapy for those with conditions worsened by stress (e.g., inflammatory bowel disease, ulcerative colitis, Crohn's disease).
  C. Massage reduces anxiety and stress of psychiatric patients.
  D. Survivors of sexual and physical abuse benefit from massage.
      1. Reduction of anxiety and stress
      2. Improved body awareness
      3. Increased ability to receive pleasurable non-sexual touch
      4. Helps patients reconnect with their bodies
      5. Helps patients experience their bodies as good

XI. Therapeutic Touch (TT)
  A. Manual therapy in which patient's energy field is rebalanced
  B. Not soft tissue manipulation, but often performed by massage practitioners
  C. Developed by nurse Dolores Kreiger in the 1970s
  D. TT technique involves
      1. Centering
      2. Placing hands in recipient's energy field to detect poor energy flow
      3. Rebalancing the energy filed using sweeping hand movements a few inches away from the skin
  E. Results in profound relaxation response that improves immune function, and allows self-healing
  F. Conditions that respond well to TT
      1. Dysfunctions of autonomic nervous system
      2. Lymphatic and circulatory dysfunctions
      3. Musculoskeletal problems
      4. Tension headaches
  G. Information on TT research available from Nurse Healers Professional Associates

XII. Complement to Chiropractic
  A. Chiropractic adjustment is a technique in which bones and joints are manipulated to return the body to proper alignment; involves forceful thrusting
  B. Massage used in context of chiropractic
      1. In preparation for an adjustment
          a. Tissues around joints more pliable
          b. Relaxation for better acceptance of touch
      2. After an adjustment
          a. Prevents tightening reaction to adjustment
          b. Helps adjustments last longer
      3. Addresses muscular problems that bring patients for adjustments
          a. Nerve constriction due to tight muscles
          b. Poor circulation
          c. Trigger points

    d. Tissue healing
    e. Pain-spasm-pain cycle
    f. Lower back pain

SUGGESTED CLASSROOM ACTIVITIES

- Analyze one or more research studies about the clinical applications of massage in more detail noting the experimental design, subjects and control group, type of massage used, results, and conclusions. Variation: Assign research studies to students for reporting to class.

- Assign different pathologies for reports and class presentations. Focus on the use of massage in the treatment of the pathology, research evidence, and goals and methods of application.

- Assign imaginary "clients" with specific pathologies to students. Have students gather relevant information, and use that information to develop a session or treatment plan for the client. Students present their plans and rationale to the class.

- Invite a panel of massage practitioners who work in medical settings to class. Ask them to comment on the clinical applications of massage in their settings and how patients respond to massage, and to answer questions from students.

- Invite a massage practitioner who specializes in working with patients with a particular pathology to class to describe their work and answer questions.

- Lead students through the process of developing scientific research related to massage and a particular pathology. Consider the research question, experimental design, subjects and control group, type of massage to use, and potential challenges in carrying out the research.

- Lead students through the process of designing a case study about the use of massage for a particular pathology. Variation: Assignment to find a person with a pathology known to respond well to massage and perform a case study.

5

Endangerment Sites, Contraindications, and Cautions

I. Introduction
   A. Most basic rule: Do no harm.
   B. Knowledge of Western anatomy and physiology are essential to ensure the safety of clients.
   C. Contraindications and endangerment sites may differ for certain forms of therapeutic massage and bodywork (e.g., Asian bodywork, energy bodywork).
   D. The information below pertains to forms of bodywork that involve soft tissue manipulation such as pressing, stroking, frictions, kneading, tapping, and vibrating, and joint movements.
   E. The information below is from the perspective of Western science.

II. Endangerment Sites [See Figure 5-1 Endangerment Sites]
   A. Anterior neck
      1. Review anatomy of anterior neck.
      2. Avoid pressure within the anterior triangle of the neck.
      3. Use light pressure on neck of the elderly, especially near major blood vessels.
   B. Vertebral column
      1. Review structure of the spine.
      2. Avoid strong pressure over spinous processes.
      3. Do not perform thrusting movements over spine.
      4. "Cracking" the back is outside of scope of massage.
   C. Thoracic cage
      1. Review structure of the thoracic cage.
      2. Avoid strong pressure over sternum, especially xiphoid process.
      3. Heavy pressure on rib cage should be avoided in elderly and those at risk for osteoporosis.
   D. Axilla
      1. Review structures in the axilla (i.e., arm pit).
      2. Avoid deep pressure on delicate structures there.
   E. Elbow
      1. Review structures around the elbow.
      2. Avoid the "funny bone" area (i.e., over the ulnar nerve).
      3. Avoid deep specific pressure over anterior surface, or fold, of the elbow.

F. Umbilicus
  1. Review structure of umbilicus (i.e., "belly button").
  2. Avoid direct heavy pressure there.
G. Kidney area
  1. Review structure and location of the kidneys.
  2. Avoid heavy percussion over the kidney area.
H. Inguinal area
  1. Review structures in the inguinal area.
  2. Avoid deep pressure in the area.
I. Popliteal fossa
  1. Review structures in popliteal area.
  2. Avoid pressure on center of this area.
J. Eyes
  1. Take care that your hand does not slip when working around the eye.
  2. Use only the lightest pressure when stroking the eyelid.
K. Major veins in extremities
  1. Review location of major veins and arteries.
  2. Apply deep effleurage on extremities moving distal to proximal.
L. General principles for safety around endangerment sites
  1. Adjust pressure to match the part of the body, condition of the tissues, and the person you are massaging.
  2. Avoid heavy pressure over nerves, blood and lymph vessels near the surface.
  3. Take care around joints where structures are less protected.
  4. If you feel a pulse, you are on a major artery. Move to a different area.
  5. If the recipient feels searing, shooting, electrical sensations, "pins and needles," numbness, you are on a nerve. Move to a different area.
  6. Any abnormal structure is a possible endangerment site. Use caution.
  7. Always work with awareness, and when in doubt, do not take a chance that might lead to injury.

III. Contraindications
  A. Definition
    1. Conditions or situations that make receiving massage inadvisable because of the harm it might do.
    2. "Any symptom or circumstance indicating inappropriateness of a form of treatment otherwise advisable."
    3. *General contraindication*—avoid the area altogether.
    4. *Regional* or *local* contraindication—avoid the immediate area.
  B. Health histories provide information about contraindications. *[See Appendix E]*
  C. Knowledge of normal anatomy and physiology, as well as pathologies is important for understanding contraindications
  D. Knowledge of pathologies reported by clients helps in session planning
  E. Principles for Contraindications and Cautions
    1. Severe distress—*Do not perform massage when the recipient is in severe distress.*
      a. Feels physically ill or nauseated
      b. Is in severe pain
      c. Has a fever
      d. Has been seriously injured recently
    2. Acute inflammation—*Do not perform massage in the presence of acute inflammation.*
      a. Any condition that ends in "itis"

      b. Appendicitis—general

      c. Rheumatoid arthritis—local

      d. Phlebitis—regional

      e. Locally inflamed tissues (red, hot, swollen, painful)—local

3. Loss of structural integrity—*Understand the physician's recommendations and the relevant anatomy and physiology in cases where there is loss of integrity in an area.*

      a. Over recent surgery

      b. Around burns

      c. Recent fracture

      d. Artificial joint replacements—obey restrictions

4. Skin conditions—*Do not touch areas of the skin where there is a pathological condition that is contagious or that may be worsened or spread by applying pressure or rubbing.*

      a. Rashes

      b. Boils

      c. Athlete's foot

      d. Herpes simplex (e.g., cold sores)

      e. Impetigo

      f. Allergies—do not use oils and lotions that client is allergic to

5. Decreased sensation—*Use extreme care in the amount of pressure used when the recipient has decreased sensation.*

      a. May be due to stroke, diabetes, spinal cord injury, medication.

      b. Recipient cannot give accurate feedback about pressure.

      c. Use extreme care in amount of pressure used.

6. Increased sensitivity to touch—*Massage only to the recipient's tolerance or comfort when there is increased sensitivity to touch.*

      a. Avoid light superficial stroking if recipient is ticklish.

7. Cardiovascular disorders—*For clients with cardiovascular system disorders, research the condition carefully, including getting a physician's recommendation if serious.*

      a. Research the condition thoroughly and follow physician's recommendations.

      b. High blood pressure—avoid circulatory massage

      c. Low blood pressure

         1. Susceptible to fainting

         2. Careful in getting up from massage table or chair

      d. Cardiac arrhythmias—avoid lateral and anterior neck

      e. Severe atherosclerosis—general contraindication

      f. Severe varicose veins—regional contraindication

      g. Stroke

         1. Recent—avoid circulatory massage

         2. Use a light pressure with blood thinner medication

8. Spreading disease by circulation—*Do not perform circulatory massage when there is a pathological condition that might spread through the lymph or cardiovascular systems.*

      a. Blood poisoning

      b. Malignant melanoma

      c. Swollen glands indicating infection

9. Bleeding and bruising—*Do not perform massage near an area where there is bleeding or bruising.*

      a. A bruise—local contraindication

      b. Acute trauma—local contraindication; general contraindication if severe

10. Edema—*Be sure of cause of edema before proceeding with massage.*

      a. General contraindications—examples

1. Inflammation due to viral infection
2. Pitted edema indicating tissue fragility
3. Lymphatic obstruction due to parasites
4. Edema due to deep vein thrombosis
5. Edema caused by cardiac, liver, kidney disease

11. Compromised immunity—*Be especially careful with personal and environmental hygiene when a recipient's immune system is suppressed.*
12. Osteoporosis—*Avoid deep pressure, heavy tapotement, and vigorous joint movement when disease is diagnosed and with those in high-risk categories.*
13. Personal appliances—Caution
    a. Contact lenses
        1. Avoid dislodging or moving lenses during face massage.
        2. Avoid pressure to eyes when recipient is prone.
        3. Taking lenses out during massage is preferable.
    b. Hearing aid
        1. Avoid dislodging during head massage.
        2. Moving ears during head massage may be annoying.
        3. Remember that recipient with hearing loss may not hear you ask for feedback or for informed consent.

IV. Medications
   A. Medications are used by an increasing number of people for a variety of ailments.
   B. Massage practitioners should be familiar with common medications, and understand the implications. *[See Table 5-1 Cautions for Massage and Medications]*
      1. Scheduling of sessions
         a. Massage *after* the client's scheduled dosage if the medication is needed for condition stability (i.e., to ensure maximum bioavailability of the medication).
            Examples: insulin-dependent diabetics, chronic pain patients, epileptic patients
         b. Massage *before* or *shortly after* the client's scheduled dosage if medication decreases the person's perception of pain or ability to give accurate feedback.
            Examples: nonsteroidal anti-inflammatory drugs, narcotic analgesics, central nervous system depressants
      2. Session length
         a. *Shorten the session* if medication causes abnormal fatigue.
            Examples: hypertension medication, antianxiety drugs, many antidepressants
         b. *Shorten the session* if the medication significantly decreases the emotional stability of the massage recipient.
            Examples: long-term corticosteroid use, medications with side-effects like mood fluctuations, anxiety, depression
      3. Selection of massage techniques
         a. For *drugs that alter clotting mechanism,* avoid heavy pressure techniques like stripping, deep kneading, cross-fiber friction.
            Examples: anticoagulants, platelet inhibitors, aspirin, anti-inflammatory drugs
         b. For *drugs that alter protective responses,* avoid deep pressure, tense-relax stretching, techniques that require accurate client feedback for safe application
            Examples: muscle relaxants, narcotic analgesics, antianxiety drugs
         c. For *drugs that compromise tissue integrity,* avoid deep pressure, heavy tapotement, forced stretching, skin rolling and wringing.
            Examples: corticosteroids

d. For *drugs that mask pain,* rely less on client feedback and more on observation and palpation to determine safe pressure.

e. For *drugs that alter a person's cooperativeness* or *that make him or her less communicative,* take time to ask questions as needed and ask for feedback.

SUGGESTED CLASSROOM ACTIVITIES

- Have students identify and touch endangerment sites on their own bodies.

- With students working in pairs, have them identify endangerment sites on each other. Variation: One student lies on a massage table supine and then prone, while the partner identifies endangerment sites.

- Provide students with an outline drawing of the body, front and back. Have them draw circles around endangerment sites, and draw and label delicate structures in the area.

- Lay an anatomical model on a massage table and lead students through the location of visceral organs and endangerment sites.

- Find an anatomy computer program that allows you strip away structures from superficial to deep. Project endangerment sites onto a screen, and strip away layers, showing the structures (e.g., nerves, blood vessels, lymph vessels, organs) in the area. Discuss the nature of the structures, their depth, and protection or lack of protection. Alternative: Do the same exercise with overheads from anatomy books.

- Invite a dermatologist to talk to the class about various skin conditions that they should be aware of and to answer questions.

- Ask students to voluntarily show skin or other structural conditions (e.g., abnormal joints) that might raise questions about contraindications or cautions when giving or receiving massage. Discuss implications for massage. Impress on students the confidential nature of this information.

- Have students practice taking health histories from each other. Each student would then present the "case" to the class as a whole and discuss the contraindications and cautions uncovered in the interview. Impress on students the confidential nature of this information. Variation 1: Have students take health histories from a family member or friend and present the case without revealing the person's identity. Variation 2: Teacher creates fictitious health histories with contraindications for presentation.

- Cut out advertisements for popular medications from magazines and newspapers. Discuss the implications for receiving massage.

- Ask students to voluntarily identify what medications they are currently taking and discuss implications for massage. Impress on students the confidential nature of this information. Variation 1: Have students take a medications inventory from a family member or friend and present the case without revealing the person's identity. Variation 2: Teacher creates fictitious medication inventories for student presentations.

6

General Principles for Giving Massage

LECTURE OUTLINE

I. The Therapeutic Relationship
  A. Involves an implicit agreement regarding the roles of the massage practitioner and the client
    1. Practitioner provides massage within scope of practice and credentials
    2. Client receives massage, participates in the therapy, fulfills obligations
  B. Professional boundaries maintain roles
    1. A limit or separation to protect the integrity of each person
    2. Includes
      a. Practicing within personal limitations
      b. Not exploiting the relationship for personal gain
      c. Limiting the impact of transference and countertransference
      d. Avoiding dual relationships
      e. Not engaging in sexual activity
      f. Respecting the client's freedom of choice and self-determination
    3. Common mistakes
      a. Going outside your area of expertise
      b. Losing the distinction between personal and professional lives
    4. Established in setting
      a. By setting itself (e.g., health care establishment policies)
      b. By the practitioner
  C. Dual relationships
    1. Any relationship besides the primary one of practitioner and client (e.g., client and friend, or client and tenant, or client and employer)
    2. Has potential to confuse roles and weaken boundaries
    3. Should be avoided if possible or entered into with caution
  D. Transference and countertransference
    1. Transference happens when a client transfers positive or negative feelings from past relationships onto the practitioner.
    2. Countertransference happens when the practitioner transfers positive or negative feelings from past relationships onto the client.
    3. Confuses past and present, and confuses the therapeutic relationship with another one.

    4. Keeping good professional boundaries and heightened awareness for the potential can limit this from happening.

II. Professional Demeanor
    A. Appearance and behavior of the practitioner
    B. Should inspire confidence and sense of safety
    C. Should help establish the professional nature of the relationship
    D. Includes several factors
        1. Clothing
            a. Be neat, clean, modest, comfortable
            b. Avoid sexually suggestive clothing
        2. Minimal jewelry
            a. No rings that scratch
            b. No dangling bracelets or necklaces
        3. Free from offensive odors
            a. Body odor: bathe, use deodorant
            b. Breath odor: use freshener
            c. Avoid strong perfume or cologne
            d. Avoid smoker odors on clothes, hands, breath
        4. Use professional language
            a. Avoid technical jargon
            b. Avoid slang
            c. Avoid sexually suggestive words and expressions
        5. Relationship should be sympathetic and understanding but not personal

III. Touching Another Person
    A. Nature of touch
        1. Touch is our most social sense.
        2. Humans have an innate touch hunger.
        3. Touch is essential for proper growth and development.
        4. Touch deprivation linked to stress, physical violence, insomnia, suppressed immune response.
    B. Touch is the primary mode of interaction in massage.
    C. Touch is more basic than technique.
        1. Touch means "to come into contact with."
        2. Touch can be physical or energetic and comes primarily through the hands of the practitioner.
        3. Holistic perspective: You touch the whole person.
        4. What may appear to be mere physical touch can have a profound effect on the mind, emotions and spirit of the receiver.
    D. Touch communicates to a sensitive receiver.
        1. Positively: Care, compassion, confidence, calmness, focus, skillfulness
        2. Negatively: Anxiety, apprehension, anger, distractedness, lack of confidence
        3. Prepare for massage by being aware of your intention to be caring and compassionate, and by becoming calm and focused.
    E. Self-care
        1. Meditation
        2. Talking to a colleague
        3. "Washing away" negative energy
    F. Touch and the therapeutic relationship
        1. Comfort levels with touch vary with cultural background

2. Maintain awareness of own and client's comfort with touch
3. Challenge is to create openness to the touch of massage
4. Be clear about the difference between friendly, caring, and affectionate touch, and sexual touch
5. Sexual touch is never appropriate in a massage setting.
6. Survivors of sexual or physical abuse and other traumatic stress especially need to feel safe and comfortable to receive the touch of massage.
7. The receiver may interpret your touch in ways unintended.
8. Clear communication and boundaries are important in a relationship based on touch.

IV. Permission to Touch
   A. There is general implicit permission to touch during massage
   B. Touching certain areas requires explicit permission to touch.
      1. Upper or inner thigh
      2. Lower abdomen
      3. Around breast tissue in women
   C. Informed consent [See Table 6-1 Elements of Informed Consent]
      1. Explain what you are going to do and where.
      2. Explain why you propose to do it (i.e., therapeutic intention).
      3. Describe what the client should expect.
      4. Ask permission to touch the area.
      5. Proceed only with explicit permission.
      6. Client has option to say no at any time.
   D. If you sense the client uncomfortable with touch, ask permission to continue.

V. Gender Considerations
   A. May be specific to a client's cultural background or the setting
   B. Factors that minimize troublesome situations related to gender
      1. Professional demeanor
      2. Good boundaries
      3. Knowledge and skill regarding touch
      4. Good verbal communication skills
   C. Cross-gender massage requires special clarity about the nonsexual nature of massage therapy.
   D. Sexualizing the therapeutic relationship is always unethical.
   E. Same-gender massage may bring up issues for some clients.
      1. If all touch is equated with sex, same-gender massage may be uncomfortable for some.
      2. Professional demeanor and boundaries help comfort levels
   F. Men should be especially mindful of women's needs for clear boundaries.

VI. Intervention Model
   A. Used if client sexualizes the relationship
   B. Seven-Step Intervention Model [See Table 6-2 Seven-Step Intervention Model]
      1. Stop the session using assertive behavior.
      2. Describe the behavior you are concerned about.
      3. Ask the client to clarify his or her behavior.
      4. Restate your intent and professional boundaries.
      5. Evaluate the client's response.
      6. Continue or discontinue the session as appropriate.
      7. Document the situation.
   C. Do not continue the session if you feel that the client is sexualizing the massage.

VII. Talking and Feedback
  A. Verbal interaction during a massage session should support the goals of the session and the needs of the receiver.
  B. For relaxation, keep talking to a minimum.
  C. People nervous about receiving massage may need more verbal interaction for direction, descriptions, and feedback.
  D. Certain techniques require frequent feedback for safety.
  E. Release of unexpressed emotions may occur (e.g., sighing or crying).
  F. Feedback to recipients about muscle tension may be useful to them.
  G. Social talking should be kept to a minimum.
     1. Exception is when social interaction is inherent in therapeutic goal.
     2. Exception may be when client needs to talk about upsetting situation.
     3. Awareness of potential for crossing boundaries should be maintained.
  H. Avoid talking to clients about your own life or troubles.
  I. Do not delve into scope of psychotherapy.

VIII. Confidentiality
  A. Ethical principle of confidentiality is based on the client's right to privacy.
  B. Includes several factors
     1. Information in health history
     2. Information told before, during, or after a session
     3. Observations about a client's condition
  C. Based on right to privacy and laws related to privacy
  D. Exceptions to the principle of confidentiality
     1. Discussion with colleague to serve client better
     2. If required by law
     3. In case of emergency
  E. See National Certification Board for Therapeutic Massage and Bodywork (NCBTMB) Standards of Practice regarding confidentiality

IX. HIPAA Privacy Rule
  A. Health Insurance Portability and Accountability Act—1996
  B. Federal standard designed to protect the medical records of individuals
  C. HIPAA Requirements
     1. Inform patients/clients about their privacy rights.
     2. Adopt and implement privacy procedures.
     3. Train employees to comply with procedures.
     4. Person designated as responsible for seeing that procedures are followed.
     5. Patients/clients able to see records, obtain copies, and ask for corrections in case of mistakes.
     6. Patient/client records secured and shown only to those that need to know their content.
     7. Patient/client must give written consent for use and disclosure of information for treatment, payment, and health care operations.
  D. Complaints handled by Health and Human Services (HHS) Office of Civil Rights

X. The Physical Environment
  A. Massage tables and chairs
     1. Features of massage table [See Figure 6-1a-b Adjustable Massage Table and Face Cradle]
        a. Height adjustable
        b. Removable, adjustable face cradle
        c. Vary in length, width, type of padding and covering
        d. Different types of practices and massage call for different table features

2. Massage chair features include seat, knee rest, armrest, chest cushion, face cradle *[See Figure 6-2a,b Adjustable Massage Chair and Position of Recipient]*
3. Improvised situations where no massage table or chair is available

B. The massage space
   1. Room temperature comfortable
      a. 75°F (24°C)
      b. Other heat sources: hot packs, electric mattress, heat lamp, blanket
   2. Air quality fresh and pleasant
      a. Well-ventilated room
      b. Allergens filtered out
   3. Lighting soft and indirect
   4. Sound peaceful and healing
      a. Avoid popular and vocal music
      b. Special music for relaxation
      c. Stimulating music for pre-event sports massage
      d. Take receiver's taste in music into consideration
      e. White noise or fish tank restful to some
      f. Silence is an option too
   5. Dressing arrangements
      a. Private and convenient
      b. Breach of professional ethics to watch clients get undressed for massage with exception of elderly and others needing help
   6. Overall cleanliness and neatness of space should be maintained
      a. Oil bottles neatly arranged and wiped clean
      b. Clean linens neatly stacked and stored away
      c. Used sheets and towels in closed containers and out of sight
      d. Floors and furniture cleaned frequently
      e. Follow local health department rules if applicable

C. Topical substances
   1. Liniment—liquid or semiliquid rubbing preparation
      a. Counterirritants
      b. Typical ingredients include camphor, menthol, turpentine
      c. Herbals include rosemary, wild majoram, cayenne pepper
      d. Rubbing too vigorously with liniments may cause blistering
      e. Are often applied after massage of an area
   2. Oils
      a. Minimizes friction for effleurage and kneading techniques
      b. Adds moisture and nutrients to skin
      c. Vegetable oils used for massage include almond, olive, grape seed, jojoba
      d. Mineral oils sometimes used
      e. Factors for choosing oils
         1. Feel of the oil (e.g., thick or thin)
         2. Inherent nutrients
         3. Scent
         4. Ease in washing out of sheets
   3. Lotions—semiliquid substances containing moisturizing substances
      a. Easily absorbed into skin
      b. Good when lubrication is desired in warm-up phase of massage, but friction is desired later
      c. More water soluble than oils, more easily washed from sheets

4. Commercial preparations available combining ingredients
5. Choose topical substances to best meet the needs of each client

XI. Safety and Comfort of the Receiver
  A. Positioning
    1. Purpose: comfort, safety and access to areas to be massaged
    2. Supine position (i.e., face up) *[See Figure 6-3 Supine Position]*
      a. Bolster under knees to take pressure off low back
      b. Neck roll for support of cervical area
    3. Prone position (i.e., face down) *[See Figure 6-4 Prone Position]*
      a. Bolster under ankles
      b. Bolster under shoulders if needed
      c. Face cradle adjusted for comfort and access *[See Figure 6-5 Face Cradle Adjustment]*
    4. Side-lying position *[See Figure 6-6 Side-Lying Position]*
      a. Support for upper leg, arm, and head
    5. Reclining (i.e., semisupine) *[See Figure 6-7 Reclining Position]*
      a. Backrest created by bolsters or hinged table
      b. Bolster under knees
  B. Draping
    1. Purpose: modesty, boundaries, warmth
    2. Avoid use of thin sheets and small towels
    3. Guidelines
      a. Genitals covered at all times
      b. Women's breasts covered (possible exception of breast massage after special training and with informed consent)
      c. Mutual consent is not acceptable reason to ignore proper draping
    4. Draping with sheet
      a. Part to be massaged is uncovered and recovered
      b. Skillful tucking enhances security of drape
      c. Examples
        1. Arm *[See Figure 6-8a–c Undraping the Arm]*
        2. Leg *[See Figure 6-9a–b Draping the Leg—Supine; Figure 6-10a–c Draping the Leg—Prone]*
        3. Women's breasts *[See Figure 6-11a–b Draping Women's Breasts]*
      d. Draping while client turns over *[See Figure 6-12 Tenting]*
        1. Do not expose client
        2. Tenting
    5. Draping with large towels is sometimes used.
    6. For some forms of massage, the client is clothed

XII. Self-Care for the Practitioner
  A. Physical self-care
    1. Hand and wrist care
      a. Nails clipped short
      b. Rings and jewelry avoided
      c. Remove offensive odors from hands
      d. Hands washed thoroughly before and after sessions
      e. Hands warm and dry for massage
      f. Preventing injury with conditioning exercises
        1. Strengthen shoulders, arms, hands and wrists
        2. Flexibility

    g. Hand mechanics
      1. Minimize strain on hands, fingers, wrists
      2. Thumb alignment *[See Figure 6-13a Correct Thumb Alignment; Figure 6–13b Incorrect Thumb Alignment]*
      3. Wrist alignment
        a. *Figure 6-14 Neutral Wrist Position*
        b. *Figure 6-15a Correct Wrist Position for Compression*
        c. *Figure 6-15b Incorrect—Pressure on Wrist*
        d. *Figure 6-15c Incorrect—Hyperextended Wrist*
      4. Use of forearm to reduce wrist strain *[See Figure 16-16 Use of Forearm for Effleurage]*
  2. Good body mechanics
    a. Proper table height *[See Figure 6-17 Determining a Good Table Height]*
    b. Keep back and neck in alignment; bend knees *[See Figure 6-18 Incorrect Alignment with Back Bent]*
    c. Use of martial arts stances for alignment and leverage
    d. Facing the head or foot of the table *[See Figure 6-19a–b Good Body Mechanics when Facing Head or Foot of Table]*
    e. Facing table directly *[See Figure 6-20a–b Good Body Mechanics when Facing Table Directly]*
    f. Sitting on a chair *[See Figure 6–21a–b Good Body Mechanics for Sitting on Chair while Performing Massage]*
  3. Avoiding strain
    a. Warm-up phase of session
    b. Use variety of techniques
    c. Use less stressful massage techniques
    d. Limit sessions scheduled per week
    e. Avoid sudden increase in number of sessions per week
    f. Scheduling guidelines
      1. Four or five 1-hour sessions maximum in one day
      2. 20 hours per week of massage total
      3. 15–20-minute breaks between sessions
      4. 30-minute break per 3 consecutive sessions
      5. Limit 4 sessions per day if strenuous type of massage
B. Emotional self-care
  1. Maintain clear professional boundaries
  2. Discuss upsetting situations with peers
  3. Seek peer and professional supervision.

XIII. Performance Elements
  A. Length of sessions
    1. Vary depending on setting and goals
    2. General health purposes—30–90 minutes, 60 minutes most common
    3. Seated massage—15–20 minutes
    4. Part of larger therapy session—10 minutes
  B. Amount of lubricant
    1. General rule: least amount of lubricant to get the job done
    2. Too much lubricant prevents good contact
    3. Too little lubricant can cause irritation
    4. Extra lubricant used for dry skin

5. Use little if any lubricant on face
6. Keep lubricant off of client's hair and clothes
7. Remove excess lubricant after massage
C. Sequence of techniques and routines
1. Deep specific techniques should be preceded by superficial warming
2. Smooth transitions between techniques add to pleasant feel
3. Routines are regular sequences of techniques performed in almost the same way each time.
a. Experienced practitioners develop routine ways of working
b. Help establish smooth patterns and are useful for learning
D. Specificity and direction
1. Much massage is applied over general areas.
2. Practitioners are said to be working with *specificity* if they focus use of their techniques (e.g., on a trigger point) or specific small area or structure (e.g., specific muscle or tendon)
3. Direction of application is expressed in anatomical terms (e.g., proximal, distal, medial, lateral)
4. Direction may be described in relation to anatomical structure (e.g., towards a muscle attachment)
5. Knowledge of anatomical structures and good palpation skills are important for specificity.
E. Pressure, rhythm, and pacing
1. Pressure
a. Pressure is related to degree of force used and compaction of tissues.
b. Pressure will vary depending on
1. Intended effect
2. Tolerance of recipient
3. Condition of tissues
c. General rule: Work from light pressure to deeper pressure to light pressure to finish.
d. Too much pressure applied too quickly can cause tissue damage.
2. Rhythm
a. A recurring pattern of movement with specific cadence, beat, or accent
b. May be smooth, flowing or uneven
c. Personal rhythm developed over time
d. Can influence effects of massage
1. Even rhythm relaxing
2. Uneven rhythm stimulating
e. Avoid breaking contact abruptly.
3. Pacing
a. Speed of application
b. Depends on desired effect
1. Slow more relaxing
2. Faster more stimulating
F. It is the skillful blending of all of these performance elements that comprise the art of massage.

SUGGESTED CLASSROOM ACTIVITIES

- Review with class NCBTMB Standards of Practice related to the therapeutic relationship.

- Create fictitious scenarios of practitioner-client situations related to maintaining professional boundaries, dual relationships, and transference and countertransference. Use for whole class or small group discussions.

- Have students role play unprofessional and professional demeanor.

- Have students evaluate themselves or each other on professional demeanor in technique classes and identify areas for improvement.

- Lead a class discussion of the students' ethnic backgrounds and their observations about the amount and comfort with touch in each group.

- Lead students through a handshake exercise. Students randomly walk around the room shaking hands with each other. Afterward discuss different kinds of handshakes and what each one seemed to communicate (e.g., confidence, shyness, competitiveness, warmth, distance). Have students practice a confident, warm, professional handshake. Variation: Practice other types of appropriate touching in professional setting (e.g., hand on shoulder or arm, hugs).

- Have students role play asking for informed consent to massage sensitive areas of the body.

- Have students role play the Seven-Step Intervention Model.

- Review information from the Health and Human Services Web site related to HIPAA rules.

- Ask table manufacturer representative or school retail manager to demonstrate features of massage tables and chairs, and critique different designs and materials.

- Demonstrate the adjustment of a massage table or chair for different practitioners and/or different clients.

- Ask students to evaluate actual massage spaces at a variety of facilities (e.g., spa, health club, rehab clinic, hospital, or at events such as health fairs and sporting events). Variables include temperature, air quality, lighting, sound, dressing arrangements, overall cleanliness, and neatness. Have students make suggestions for improvement.

- Bring a variety of topical substances to class and have students evaluate them in terms of their quality and usefulness for massage.

- Have students practice positioning each other in supine, prone, side-lying, and reclining positions using appropriate bolsters.

- Have students practice draping skills with a sheet, uncovering and covering body regions as if they were giving massage. Partners give feedback and critique. Variations: Groups of three with giver, receiver, observer; use large towels.

- Teach students a short tai chi sequence to practice stances and weight transfer.

7

Western Massage Techniques

LECTURE OUTLINE

I. Overview of Western Massage
  A. Basis of most massage therapy performed in North America and Europe today
    1. Commonly found in spas, health clubs, private practice
    2. Foundation of therapeutic applications in professions of massage therapy, physical therapy, athletic training, and nursing
  B. Origins in work of Ling of Sweden and Metzger of Amsterdam, and later Kellogg, McMillan and others *[See Chapter 2 for more on history]*
  C. Based on Western science and understanding of health and disease
  D. Major effects include improving circulation, general relaxation, muscle relaxation, joint mobility, and promoting healthy skin *[See Chapters 3 and 4 for more on effects of massage]*
  E. Western massage technique categories *[See Figure 1-2 Seven Basic Western Technique Categories; and CD-ROM Video]*
    1. Effleurage
    2. Petrissage
    3. Friction
    4. Tapotement
    5. Vibration
    6. Touch without movement
    7. Joint movements

II. Western Massage Techniques
  A. Effleurage techniques slide or glide over the skin with a smooth continuous motion *[See CD-ROM Video Effleurage Segment]*
    1. Pressure used varies from light to deep
    2. Uses of effleurage
      a. Begin a session
      b. Apply oil or lotion
      c. Accustom receiver to touch of practitioner
      d. Warming technique
      e. Connecting and transition technique
      f. Fluid circulation
      g. Break from more specific techniques

    h. Conclude work on an area or end the session
  3. Qualities of pressure, pacing, and rhythm can be varied for different effects. Examples:
    a. Effleurage applied on the back with moderate pressure, slow and smooth can evoke the relaxation response
    b. Effleurage applied to the limbs with moderate to deep pressure moving distal to proximal can enhance venous return
    c. Deep effleurage can provide a passive stretch to a muscle group
  4. Variations of effleurage
    a. Basic sliding effleurage *[See Figures 7-1, 7-2, 7-3]*
    b. Thumb stripping *[See Figure 7-4]*
    c. Shingles effleurage *[See Figure 7-5]*
    d. Bilateral tree stroking *[See Figure 7-6]*
    e. Three-count stroking of trapezius *[See Figure 7-7]*
    f. Horizontal stroking *[See Figure 7-8]*
    g. Mennell's superficial stroking *[See Figure 7-9]*
    h. Nerve strokes
    i. Knuckling effleurage *[See Figure 7-10]*

B. <u>Petrissage</u> techniques lift, wring, or squeeze soft tissues in a kneading motion, or press or roll the tissues under or between the hands. *[See CD-ROM Video Petrissage Segment]*
  1. Performed with one or two hands depending on size of area
  2. Minimal sliding over the skin
  3. Uses and effects of petrissage
    a. "Milk" a muscle of accumulated waste products
    b. Increase local circulation
    c. Assist venous return
    d. Separate muscle fibers
    e. Evoke muscle relaxation
  4. Before performing deep petrissage, warm the area
  5. Avoid using too much pressure which can pinch or bruise tissues
  6. Adjust pressure for the individual and tissue condition
  7. Variations of petrissage
    a. Basic two-handed kneading *[See Figure 7-11]*
    b. One-handed kneading *[See Figure 7-12]*
    c. Alternating one-hand kneading *[See Figure 7-13]*
    d. Circular two-handed petrissage *[See Figure 7-14]*
    e. Alternating fingers-to-thumb petrissage *[See Figure 7-15]*
    f. Skin rolling *[See Figure 7-16]*
    g. Compression using reinforced palm *[See Figure 7-17]*
    h. Rolling

C. <u>Friction</u> techniques are performed by rubbing one surface over another repeatedly. *[See CD-ROM Video Friction Segment]*
  1. Superficial friction or skin rubbing creates heat and stimulates
    a. Examples of superficial friction
      1. Using the knuckles *[See Figure 7-18]*
      2. With sawing motion *[See Figure 7-19]*
  2. Deep friction moves the skin over deeper tissues
    a. Addresses smaller area for more specificity
    b. Performed cross-fiber, parallel, or circular
    c. Uses of deep friction
      1. To break tissue adhesions

       2. To create movement in tissues around joints

       3. To massage in small spaces like suboccipital region

       4. To massage areas that lack muscle bulk such as the head

    d. Examples of deep friction

       1. Circular friction around knee *[See Figure 7-20]*

       2. Cross-fiber friction to paraspinals *[See Figure 7-21]*

       3. Circular friction to IT band *[See Figure 7-22]*

    e. Friction used in rehabilitation

       1. Deep transverse (Cyriax) friction *[See Figure 7-23]*

       2. Applied directly to site of lesion

       3. Uses of deep transverse friction

          a. Facilitate healthy scar formation

          b. Separation of fibers

          c. Breaks adhesions

       4. Cyriax principles for applying deep friction

          a. Fingers and skin move together over deeper tissues

          b. Effect more important than amount of pressure

          c. Applied over precise site of the lesion

          d. Tissue must be in appropriate tension

          e. 6 to 12 sessions of 20 minutes each on alternate days for best results

D. <u>Tapotement</u> consists of a series of brisk percussive movements following each other in rapid, alternating fashion. *[See CD-ROM Video Tapotement Segment]*

  1. Has stimulating effect and is pleasant to receive if done skillfully

  2. Performance principles

    a. Movement is rapid, light, and rhythmic.

    b. Hands should bounce off the surface lightening the impact.

    c. The sound itself can be pleasing and therapeutic.

    d. Different hand positions create different sensations and sounds.

    e. Rhythms can vary for different effects.

    f. Vary force used with area receiving the technique.

       1. Example: light force on the head

       2. Example: the back can usually take more force

  3. Uses of tapotement

    a. Finishing a section, side of the body, or the session itself

    b. To increase alertness and mental clarity

    c. For athletes before competition

  4. Variations of tapotement

    a. Hacking *[See Figure 7-24]*

    b. Rapping *[See Figure 7-25]*

    c. Cupping *[See Figure 7-26]*

    d. Clapping

    e. Slapping

    f. Tapping *[See Figure 7-27]*

    g. Pincement *[See Figure 7-28]*

    h. Quacking *[See Figure 7-29]*

    i. Squishes

E. <u>Vibration</u> is an oscillating, quivering, or trembling motion; or movement back and forth or up and down performed quickly and repeatedly. *[See CD-ROM Video Vibration Segment]*

  1. Types of vibration

    a. Fine vibration is applied in a small area with fingertips

b. Coarse vibration involves shaking a muscle belly
2. Uses of vibration
   a. Over abdomen to stimulate digestive organs
   b. Jostling to raise awareness of tension in muscles
   c. Increase circulation and muscle relaxation
   d. Have stimulating effect on tissues
   e. Numb or relax specific muscles
3. Electric vibrators may be used for fine vibration *[See Figure 7-30]*
4. Variations of vibration
   a. Fine vibration over abdomen *[See Figure 7-31]*
   b. Effleurage with light vibration
   c. Shaking—course vibration *[See Figure 7-32]*
   d. Jostling—course vibration *[See Figure 7-33]*

F. Touch without movement involves touch but without any visible movement. *[See CD-ROM Video Touch without Movement Segment]*
   1. Not casual or social touch, but skilled touch with intention
   2. Passive touch is simply laying the fingers, one hand, or both hands lightly on the body.
      a. Effects
         1. Imparts heat to an area
         2. Has a calming influence on nervous system
         3. Some believe that it helps balance energy
      b. Uses
         1. Begin or end a massage session
         2. Transition before recipient changes position
      c. Examples
         1. Holding the head *[See Figure 7-34]*
         2. Holding the feet *[See Figure 7-35]*
   3. Direct pressure, aka direct static pressure, is applied with a thumb, finger, knuckle, or elbow.
      a. Also considered "static friction" or a form of compression
      b. *Ischemic compression* is a form of direct pressure applied with enough force to cause blanching.
         1. Vasodilation upon release of pressure
         2. Used to deactivate trigger points *[See Chapter 13 Neuromuscular Therapy]*
      c. Application guidelines
         1. Precede by warming the area.
         2. Apply slowly and carefully.
         3. Follow up with smoothing techniques.
         4. Application variables include intention, amount of pressure used, locations of areas pressed, and duration of pressure.
      d. Examples
         1. Direct pressure to suboccipital muscles *[See Figure 7-36]*
         2. Ischemic compression *[See Figure 7-37]*
      e. Uses of direct pressure
         1. Relieve pain
         2. Diminish congestion in tissues
         3. Helps muscles relax
      f. Related theories
         1. Zone therapy
         2. Motor points

3. Stress points
4. Reflexology points
5. Trigger points
6. Acupressure points

SUGGESTED CLASSROOM ACTIVITIES

- Show CR-ROM video segments on Western massage along with lecture.

- Demonstrate Western massage techniques on a receiver along with lecture. Variation: Use video camera for close-up view for large groups.

- Alternate lecture with hands-on practice of each technique category.

- Once basic information has been presented, demonstrate different techniques without talking and ask students to describe the action in detail. Variation: Students list the effects as well.

- Demonstrate different forms of therapeutic massage and bodywork. Ask students to describe the techniques using Western massage categories and to identify any techniques that do not fit into those categories. Discuss differences in intention and application of different forms. Variation: Invite guests to demonstrate different forms; or show videos of different forms. Conduct student discussion as described previously.

- Demonstrate technique variations for each Western massage category and ask students to identify, compare, and contrast their effects.

- Demonstrate technique applications varying the performance elements (e.g., rhythm, pacing, direction) and ask students to discuss potential differences in their effects. [See Chapter 6 General Principles for Giving Massage]

- Demonstrate different massage techniques and ask students to comment about ways to maintain good body mechanics while performing them. [See Chapter 6 General Principles for Giving Massage]

- Show a video of a full-body Western massage. Ask students to name techniques as they are being performed, and the likely intention of the practitioner.

- For massage therapy programs: Invite a physical therapist to class to demonstrate how massage techniques are used in their practices. Variation: Invite a nurse to demonstrate massage as used in his or her practice; invite a respiratory therapist to demonstrate massage techniques used in respiratory care.

8

Joint Movements

LECTURE OUTLINE

I. Categories of Joint Movements
   A. *Free active movements* are performed without assistance from practitioner.
   B. In *assisted movements* a practitioner helps the movement in some way.
   C. In *resisted movements* the practitioner offers resistance.
   D. During *passive movements* the recipient remains totally relaxed.
   E. *Mobilizing techniques,* or joint mobilizations in the context of massage therapy, are passive movements performed within the normal range of joint movement.
      1. Nonspecific movements of joints and surrounding soft tissues
      2. Can be easily integrated into a massage session
   F. *Stretching* is a type of passive joint movement performed to the limit of range of motion, with a slight stretch or lengthening beyond that point.
      1. Used to increase flexibility
      2. Used for muscle relaxation
   G. *Joint manipulations* or *adjustments* are *not* within the scope of massage therapy.
      1. Specific attempts to realign a misaligned joint usually with thrusting
      2. Cracking necks and backs, and popping toes should *not* be performed as part of standard Western massage

II. Uses of Joint Movements
   A. Stretch surrounding soft tissues
   B. Increase range of motion and flexibility
   C. Stimulate production of synovial fluid
   D. Increase kinesthetic awareness
   E. Stimulate muscle relaxation
   F. Build muscle strength (i.e., resisted movements)
   G. Improve posture and body alignment
   H. With athletes
      1. Improving performance
      2. Preventing injury
      3. For rehabilitation
   I. Basic technique of Trager Psychophysical Integration®

J. Teach recipients to let go of tension

K. Provide a kinetic dimension to a massage session

III. General Principles for Joint Movements

A. Practitioners should be knowledgeable about muscle and joint anatomy and about normal range of joint motion to help prevent injuries.

B. Caution advised with certain conditions

1. Abnormality of joint and bony structures
2. Hypermobility at a joint
3. Recent injury related to the joint or surrounding soft tissue
4. Joint diseases such as bursitis and arthritis
5. Scarring, shortening, loss of muscle due to past injury
6. "Hardware" such as metal pins and plates
7. Joint replacements
8. Massage contraindicated around inflammation

C. Palpation skills useful for assessment

1. Can detect condition of movement at a joint
   a. Movement restrictions
   b. Areas of tightness
   c. Patterns of holding
   d. Limits of range of motion in stretches
2. *Drag* refers to resistance felt as soft tissues around a joint are stretched.
3. *End feel* refers to resistance felt as limit of a stretch is approached.

D. *Static stretches* are passive joint movements performed by moving the parts to be stretched into position and holding for 10–15 seconds at the limit of movement.

1. Move in a slow controlled manner feeling for the point of resistance.
2. Avoid sudden, forceful, or bouncing movements.
3. Use feedback from the recipient to avoid over stretching.
4. After initial stretch (10–15 seconds), try to increase the stretch further.
5. Stretch for limit of 30–45 seconds overall.
6. Ease the joint out of the stretched position.

E. *Contract-relax-stretch* (CRS) is a stretch facilitation technique.

1. Steps in CRS
   a. Get the joint into position for the stretch.
   b. Ask the recipient to contract the muscle to be stretched against your resistance (resisted movement) for about 10 seconds.
   c. Ask the recipient to relax, and take a deep breath in.
   d. As they breathe out, apply the stretch.
2. Rest for a few seconds before applying again.

F. Reciprocal inhibition is another stretch facilitation technique.

1. Steps in reciprocal inhibition
   a. Get the joint into position for the stretch.
   b. Ask the recipient to contract the target muscle's *antagonist* against a resistance for about 10 seconds.
   c. Ask the recipient to relax, and take a deep breath in.
   d. As they breathe out, apply the stretch.
2. The target muscle (agonist) relaxes as its antagonist contracts.

G. Breathing is used to help the recipient relax for optimal stretching.

1. The body is more relaxed during the exhalation phase of breathing.
2. Holding the breath causes tension in the musculature and restricts movement.

3. Just before applying a stretch, ask the recipient to "take a deep breath in" and then "breathe out slowly."
4. As they exhale, apply the stretch.
   H. Summary of guidelines for applying stretches
   1. Stay within the normal range of motion of the joint.
   2. Qualities for mobilizing joints are smooth, free, and loose.
   3. Warm surrounding soft tissues before applying a stretch.
   4. Use breathing to enhance a stretch.
   5. Stay within the comfort range of the recipient.
   6. Be aware of joint abnormalities and adapt movements accordingly.

IV. Joint Movement Techniques *[See CD-ROM Video Segment on Joint Movements]*
   A. Neck
   1. Structure and movement in the neck
      a. Seven cervical vertebrae and surrounding soft tissues
      b. Vertebrae are stacked vertically with an anterior convex curve.
      c. Neck movements
         1. Flexion
         2. Extension
         3. Hyperextension
         4. Lateral flexion
         5. Rotation
   2. Mobilizing techniques for the neck
      a. Move the neck through its full range of motion.
      b. *Finger push-ups* produce a gentle neck movement.
      c. *Meltdown* is a variation of finger push-ups in suboccipital area.
      d. *Wavelike movement* created with deep effleurage *[See Figure 9-21]*
   3. Stretches for the neck
      a. Lateral flexion *[See Figure 8-1]*
      b. Neck rotation to left and right.
      c. Cross-arm stretch in forward flexion *[See Figure 8-2]*
      d. Cross-arm stretch with head rotated
   B. Shoulder girdle
   1. Structure and movement in shoulder girdle
      a. Includes the gleno-humeral, acromio-clavicular, and scapulo-clavicular joints.
      b. Shoulder girdle movements
         1. Upper arm
            a. Flexion
            b. Extension
            c. Hyperextension
            d. Abduction
            e. Adduction
            f. Rotation
            g. Horizontal flexion
         2. Scapulae
            a. Elevation
            b. Depression
            c. Upward and downward rotation and tilt
            d. Retraction and protraction
   3. Entire shoulder can perform circumduction

2. Mobilizing techniques for the shoulder girdle
 a. Wagging the arm *[See Figure 8-3]*
 b. Shaking the arm *[See Figure 8-4]*
 c. Passive shoulder roll—supine *[See Figure 8-5]*
 d. Scapula mobilizing—prone *[See Figure 8-6]*
3. Stretches for the shoulder girdle
 a. Horizontal flexion *[See Figure 8-7]*
 b. Overhead stretch *[See Figure 8-8]*
 c. Overhead stretch in massage chair *[See Figure 8-9]*

C. Elbow
1. Structure and movement of the elbow
 a. Junction of distal end of humerus and proximal ends of radius and ulna.
 b. Movements at the elbow
  1. Flexion and extension of forearm
  2. Pronation and supination of forearm
2. Mobilizing techniques for the elbow
 a. Wagging the arm *[See Figure 8-3]*
 b. Pronate and supinate the forearm
 c. Circling the forearm *[See Figure 8-10]*
3. Stretches for the elbow
 a. Overhead stretch *[See Figure 8-8]*
 b. Straightening the arm for shortened biceps

D. Wrist
1. Structure and movement at the wrist
 a. Formed by union of the carpal bones with the distal end of the radius and midcarpal joint
 b. Movements at the wrist
  1. Flexion
  2. Extension
  3. Hyperextension
  4. Radial and ulnar deviation (side-to-side)
  5. Circumduction
2. Mobilizing techniques for the wrist
 a. Move hand through full range of motion, fingers interwoven with recipient's fingers—supine.
 b. Waving
3. Stretches at the wrist
 a. Hyperextending the wrist; stretches forearm flexors *[See Figure 8-11]*
 b. Flexion at the wrist; stretches forearm extensors *[See Figure 8-12]*

E. Hand
1. Structure and movement of the hand
 a. Complex structure with many joints.
 b. Movements of the hand
  1. Fingers: flexion, extension, abduction, adduction
  2. Grasping and holding objects
2. Mobilizing techniques for the hand
 a. Figure-eights at knuckles *[See Figure 8-13]*
 b. Scissoring of metacarpals *[See Figure 8-14]*
3. Stretches for the hands
 a. Hyperextend fingers at the knuckles

      b. Hyperextend hand at knuckles and wrist *[See Figure 8-11]*

      c. Flexion at the wrist *[See Figure 8-12]*

F. Chest

  1. Structure and movement of the chest

      a. Area on the front and sides of the trunk defined by the ribs, sternum, and clavicle

      b. Moves with exhalation and inhalation of breathing

      c. Site of shoulder and arm muscle attachments

  2. Mobilizing techniques for the chest

      a. Gentle rib cage rocking—from one side *[See Figure 8-15]*

      b. Gentle rib cage rocking—from both sides *[See Figure 8-16]*

  3. Stretches for the chest

      a. Limited by structure

      b. Overhead stretch *[See Figure 8-8]*

G. Hip

  1. Structure and movement at the hip

      a. Hip joint is a ball and socket joint.

      b. Movements at the hip

         1. Flexion

         2. Extension

         3. Hyperextension

         4. Abduction

         5. Adduction

         6. Diagonal abduction and adduction

         7. Outward and inward rotation

         8. Circumduction

  2. Mobilizing techniques for the hip

      a. Rocking the leg into rotation *[See Figure 8-17]*

      b. Move the hip through its full range *[See Figure 8-18]*

  3. Stretches for the hip

      a. Knee to chest—supine *[See Figure 8-19]*

      b. Straight leg flexion *[See Figure 8-20]*

      c. Diagonal adduction of the thigh *[See Figure 8-21]*

      d. Stretch into hyperextension—side-lying *[See Figure 8-22]*

H. Knee

  1. Structure and movement at the knee

      a. Hinge joint formed by articulation of femur and tibia

      b. Patella or knee cap embedded in connective tissues

      c. Movements at the knee

         1. Flexion

         2. Extension

         3. Minor inward and outward rotation of the tibia possible

  2. Mobilizing techniques for the knee (all in prone position)

      a. Wagging by lifting bent leg at the ankle with movement back and forth

      b. Leg toss by "throwing" the bent lower leg from hand to hand

      c. Circling the lower leg

  3. Stretches at the knee

      a. Straight leg stretches also stretch muscles that cross the knee *[See Figure 8-20]*

      b. Heel of foot toward buttocks—prone *[See Figure 8-23]*

I. Ankle

  1. Structure and movement at the ankle

      a. Hinge joint formed by junction of talus with malleoli of the tibia and fibula

      b. Movements at the ankle

         1. Dorsiflexion (flexion)

         2. Plantar flexion (extension)

         3. Pronation (eversion and abduction)

         4. Supination (inversion and adduction)

  2. Mobilizing techniques for the ankle

      a. Mobilizing with dorsiflexion—prone *[See Figure 8-24]*

      b. Passive movement through full range—prone

  3. Stretches at the ankle

      a. Stretch in dorsiflexion

      b. Stretch in plantarflexion *[See Figure 8-25]*

J. Foot

  1. Structure and movement

      a. Elastic arched structure made up of 26 bones and designed for support and propulsion

      b. Movements of the foot

         1. Gliding between irregular intertarsal joints

         2. Flexion and extension of toes

         3. Spreading of the toes

  2. Mobilizing techniques for the foot—supine

      a. Figure-eights at knuckles *[Similar to Figure 8-13]*

      b. Scissoring of metatarsals *[Similar to Figure 8-14]*

      c. Effleurage on underside of toes for mobilizing into extension—especially for curled toes (i.e., shortened flexors)

  3. Stretches for the foot

      a. Plantarflex the foot into a stretch

      b. Dorsiflex the foot into a stretch

      c. Lateral stretch pulling sides of foot *[See Figure 8-26]*

      d. Interlocking fingers between toes *[See Figure 8-27]*

SUGGESTED CLASSROOM ACTIVITIES

- Show CD-ROM video segment on joint movements in conjunction with the lecture.

- Review joint structures in detail using anatomical models, instructional videos, computer anatomy programs, and other instructional aides.

- Lead students through a review of movements possible at each joint (e.g. flexion, extension, rotation, etc.) using their own bodies for active movements and working in partners or groups of three for passive movements.

- Demonstrate joint mobilizing techniques and stretches on a receiver in conjunction with the lecture. Variation: Use video camera for close-up view for large groups.

- Invite a practitioner of Trager Psychophysical Integration® to class to demonstrate this form of bodywork. Discuss intent, variety, and quality of the joint movements. Variation: Show a video about Trager bodywork and/or Mentastics®.

- Place a skeletal model on a massage table to demonstrate joint movement during mobilizing techniques and stretches.

- Alternate lecture on each body section or joint with hands-on practice of techniques.

- After anatomy review of each body section or joint, have students explore different joint mobilizing techniques expanding on the examples given in the text.

- Demonstrate a stretch (e.g., straight leg flexion—supine) using static stretch, contract-relax-stretch, and reciprocal inhibition. Compare degree of stretch accomplished with each method. Variation: Use a goniometer for more exact measurement of degree of flexibility.

- Have students practice static stretch, contract-relax-stretch, and reciprocal inhibition for stretches on different parts of the body.

- Lead students through a full-body session on a massage table using mainly mobilizing and stretching techniques. Recipients remain clothed with no draping.

- Supervise practice of full-body massage session with students incorporating some mobilizing and stretching techniques on different body areas. *[See Chapter 9 Full-Body Western Massage, and Chapter 10 Regional Applications]*

9

Full-Body Western Massage

LECTURE OUTLINE

I. Overview
    A. Full-body Western massage sessions last from 30 to 90 minutes.
    B. Purpose includes both general health and therapeutic goals.
        1. Improving circulation
        2. Relaxing muscles
        3. Improving joint mobility
        4. Eliciting the relaxation response
        5. Promoting healthy skin
        6. Creating sense of well-being
        7. Addressing therapeutic needs
    C. Includes techniques from the seven Western massage categories
    D. Typically uses oil or lotion
    E. Practitioners combine and blend techniques in their unique styles

II. General Guidelines
    A. Draping with sheet or large towel for warmth and modesty
        1. Genitals covered at all times
        2. Women's breasts covered
    B. Sequence of body regions for routine approach
        1. Alternate supine, prone, and side-lying positions
        2. Sequence should facilitate smooth flow from region to region
        3. Move clockwise around the table
        4. Starting point, direction (e.g., clockwise), endpoint
        5. Example of sequence with start in prone position
            a. Start on back, buttocks, legs
            b. Turn to supine
            c. Legs, feet, arms, shoulders
            d. Neck, chest, abdomen
            e. Ending with head and face
        6. Example of sequence with start in supine position
            a. Start on head and face, neck

      b. Shoulders, arms, hands

      c. Chest and abdomen

      d. Legs and feet

      e. Turn to prone

      f. Legs and buttocks

      g. Ending with the back

    7. Advantages in starting prone or supine

      a. Starting prone

        1. Feels safe to someone new to massage

        2. Back massage triggers relaxation response sooner

        3. Recipient more alert ending face up

      b. Starting supine gives head and neck priority, which is important for those working at desks or who experience eye or neck strain in their work or leisure activities.

C. Order of techniques on specific body region

    1. *Undrape* the body region to be massaged.

    2. Perform *opening and warming techniques.*

      a. Effleurage

        1. To apply oil or lotion

        2. To warm the area

        3. To increase circulation

      b. Compression can be used for opening if recipient is clothed.

    3. *Combination of techniques* for health promotion (effleurage, petrissage, warming friction and joint movements).

      a. Improve circulation

      b. Relax muscles

      c. For general relaxation

      d. Improve joint mobility

    4. *More specific massage* as needed (e.g., deep friction, vibration, direct pressure, stretches)

    5. *Transition techniques* provide continuity and flow

    6. *Finishing techniques* reconnect, sedate, stimulate, signal finish.

      a. Effleurage and tapotement help reconnect

      b. Light effleurage or nerve strokes are soothing

      c. Tapotement is stimulating

      d. Passive touch (e.g., holding feet or head) is calming.

    7. Redrape when finished.

D. Continuity and flow

    1. Create a sense of continuous touch throughout the session.

    2. Do not remove hands abruptly after establishing contact.

    3. Sense of flow achieved through orderly sequence and smooth transitions.

    4. Skillful draping important for smooth transitions.

E. Rhythm, pacing, specificity in full-body massage

    1. Rhythm is smooth and even.

    2. Pacing is moderate.

      a. Half hour full-body massage has faster pace with less attention to detail.

      b. General relaxation session will be slower paced with fewer specific and stimulating techniques.

      c. Specific massage in one area shortens time and detail in other areas.

III. Full-Body Massage Routine

A. Practitioners develop their own styles and routine ways of working.

B. Elements of a full-body routine *[See Table 9-1 Summary of the Elements of a Full-Body Western Massage Routine]*
   1. Regular starting point and opening techniques
   2. Specific sequence of body regions
   3. Certain order of techniques in each body region
   4. Regular way of ending the session
C. Routines typically evolve with further training and experience
D. Routines are modified to meet the individual recipient's needs
E. *Eclectic practitioners* integrate other forms of massage and bodywork with Western massage

IV. Example of One-Hour Full-Body Western Massage Session
   A. Prone position (25 minutes)
      1. Back (15 minutes)
         a. Uncover back to the waist.
         b. Bilateral tree stroking to apply oil *[Figure 7-6]*
         c. Shingles effleurage along one side of back *[Figure 7-5]*
         d. Circular friction along erector muscles *[See Figure 7-21]*
         e. Apply deeper pressure with circular friction *[See Figure 9-1]*
         f. Deep effleurage with thumb along lower back (Variation: knuckling friction) *[See Figure 7-18]*
         g. Deep effleurage over back and shoulder *[See Figure 9-2]*
         h. Two-handed petrissage over entire back *[See Figure 7-14]*
         i. Kneading upper trapezius *[See Figure 9-3]*
         j. Three-count stroking of trapezius *[See Figure 7-7]*
         k. Horizontal stroking from lower back to shoulders *[See Figure 7-8]*
         l. Light effleurage to finish the side, walk to other side
         m. Repeat c thru l to the other side of the back.
         n. Redrape the back.
         o. Finish entire back with light tapotement.
      2. Lower limbs and buttocks (10 minutes)
         a. Undrape the right leg to the waist. *[See Figure 6-10a–c]*
         b. Basic effleurage to apply oil to entire area *[See Figure 9-4]*
         c. Warm buttocks muscles using deep circular effleurage *[See Figure 9-5]*
         d. Perform compressions on buttocks with the fist.
         e. Repeat circular effleurage on buttocks.
         f. Two to three long effleurage stokes to entire leg for transition
         g. Deep effleurage with fists to hamstring muscles *[See Figure 9-6]*
         h. Horizontal stroking to upper leg
         i. Two-handed kneading of upper leg muscles *[See Figure 9-7]*
         j. Transition with effleurage first to upper then to entire leg
         k. Two-handed kneading of lower leg muscles
         l. Finish side with a few light effleurage strokes to entire leg/hip
         m. Recover leg and walk to other side
         n. Repeat a thru m on other leg
         o. Gentle rocking to finish entire back side
      3. Ask the recipient to turn over, use tent draping *[See Figure 6-12]*
   B. Supine Position (35 minutes)
      1. Lower limbs (10 minutes)
         a. Uncover left leg. *[See Figure 6-10a–c]*

b. Basic effleurage to apply oil to entire leg
c. Deep effleurage to thigh
d. Two-handed kneading of thigh
e. Jostling of thigh *[See Figure 9-8]*
f. Transition with effleurage to entire leg, then just to lower.
g. Circular friction around knee with heels of hands *[See Figure 9-9]*
h. Thumb stripping to tibialis anterior *[See Figure 9-10]*
i. Direct pressure along tibialis anterior *[See Figure 9-11]*
j. Circular friction around ankle with fingertips
k. Mobilize ankle using heels of hands. *[See Figure 9-12]*
l. Effleurage to foot and between metatarsals *[See Figure 7-2]*
m. Slide along bottom of foot with fist. *[See Figure 9-13]*
n. Slapping tapotement to bottom of foot using back of hand
o. Finish entire leg with long effleurage strokes, recover leg
p. Repeat a thru o on right leg.
q. Nerve strokes over draped legs as transition

2. Arms and shoulders (10 minutes)
a. Uncover right arm and shoulder. *[See Figure 6-8a–c]*
b. Effleurage to apply oil to entire arm.
c. Alternating petrissage to upper arm *[See Figure 7-13]*
d. Passive shoulder roll *[See Figure 8-5]*
e. Transition with light effleurage to entire arm.
f. Deeper effleurage to lower arm.
g. Knead muscles of lower arm.
h. Thumb stripping to flexors and extensors *[See Figure 9-14]*
i. Transition with effleurage to entire arm.
j. Interlock fingers with recipient, and mobilize hand at knuckles
k. Mobilize wrist through range of motion.
l. Effleurage to back of hand, gently squeeze each finger.
m. Effleurage to palm of hand *[See Figure 9-15]*
n. Transition with effleurage to shoulders.
n. Effleurage with loose fist to pectoral muscles. *[See Figure 9-16]*
o. Effleurage over sternum with palm. *[See Figure 9-17]*
p. Finish arm with long effleurage strokes and redrape.
q. Repeat a–p on left arm and shoulder.

3. Abdomen (5 minutes)
a. Ask permission to massage the abdomen.
b. Undrape for abdominal massage. *[For women—See Figure 6-11]*
c. Passive touch on abdomen to establish contact
d. Light to moderate effleurage in clockwise circular pattern *[See Figure 9-18]*
e. Fine fingertip vibration moving clockwise around abdomen *[See Figure 7-31]*
f. Wavelike petrissage with flat palm
g. Transition with circular effleurage.
h. Horizontal stroking over waist and abdomen
i. Passive touch to finish
j. Recover with drape.

4. Neck and shoulders (5 minutes)
a. Sit at head of table. *[See Figure 6-21]*
b. Mobilize shoulders with "cat paw" movement. *[See Figure 9-19]*

    c. Apply lubricant to both sides of neck with effleurage.

    d. Turn head slightly to left to perform effleurage from shoulder to occiput with loose fist. *[See Figure 9-20]*

    e. Circular friction along posterior cervical muscles

    f. Stripping posterior cervical muscles

    g. Repeat d–f on right side.

    h. Wavelike mobilizing technique to neck *[See Figure 9-21]*

    i. Finish with effleurage to both sides of the neck.

5. Face and head (5 minutes)

    a. Use very little or no lubricant on face and head.

    b. Passive touch on face

    c. Gentle effleurage with palms from jaw to temples *[See Figure 9-22]*

    d. Circular friction over masseter and temporalis muscles

    e. Stroke forehead using thumbs—medial to lateral

    f. Circular petrissage with thumbs to forehead
      [Similar to Figure 7-14]

    g. Stroke alongside of nose and under cheekbones.

    h. Light direct pressure under cheekbones

    i. Circular friction over scalp

    j. Finish entire session with holding the head. *[See Figure 9-23]*

SUGGESTED CLASSROOM ACTIVITIES

- Demonstrate massage of each section of the body, describing techniques as performed.

- Talk students through practice massage of each section of the body, and then through the entire routine timing them to minutes allotted.

- Invite two to three professional massage therapists to demonstrate their approaches to a particular part of the body (e.g., the legs or the back). Discuss differences and similarities in approaches.

- Once students know a foundation routine, have them experiment with using different techniques and combinations using the basic elements of beginning, warming phase, technique combinations, transitions, and finishing techniques.

- Lead students through a 30 minute full-body session with specified timing for each section.

- Have students experiment with a 90-minute full-body massage session, adding specificity to each section as described in Chapter 10 Regional Applications.

10

Regional Applications

I. Overview
   A. Reasons for giving more time and attention to a specific body region
      1. Recipient request
      2. Practitioner observation and assessment
      3. Information from health history form
      4. Referral from health care provider
      5. Prescription for treatment
   B. Wholeness of the person
      1. The interconnectedness or wholeness of the body should always be kept in mind when giving massage.
      2. Massage in a specific area will necessarily flow into surrounding regions and sometimes to the entire body.
   C. Meaning of body regions
      1. Each body region has meaning for the recipient in human terms.
         a. What it allows us to be and to do in this world
         b. Social and emotional associations
         c. Special significance in a person's life (e.g., musician's hands)
      2. During massage, you are not just touching a body, you are touching a person.

II. Regional Applications
   A. Head and face
      1. Meaning
         a. Human consciousness
         b. Center for thinking and processing information
         c. Senses housed in head (i.e., sight, hearing, taste, smell)
         d. Communication through speech
         e. Facial expressions convey feelings and meaning
         f. Furrowed brows and frowns of concentration
         g. Holding mental and emotional stress
      2. Applications of massage
         a. Release tension in head and face from work or leisure activities.

      b. Release tension from emotional distress, worry, anxiety.
      c. Relax related to clenching teeth.
      d. Release tension caused by holding back emotions.
      e. In treatment for pathologies such as Bell's palsy and stroke.
   3. Review musculature of face and head.
      a. Muscles of expression *[See Figure 10-1]*
      b. Muscles of mastication
      c. Muscles of movement
   4. Techniques to integrate into head and face massage
      a. Squeeze to eyebrows *[See Figure 10-2]*
      b. Effleurage over eyelids *[See Figure 10-3]*
      c. Thumb slides along the nose *[See Figure 10-4]*
      d. Direct pressure along zygomatic arch *[See Figure 10-5]*
      e. Massage around mouth and jaw *[See Figure 10-6]*
      f. Massaging the ears *[See Figures 10-7 and 10-8]*
      g. Mobilizing the scalp *[See Figure 10-9]*
      h. Circular friction to muscles on the head
      i. Passive touch over eyes *[See Figure 10-10]*
      j. Pressing sides of head *[See Figure 10-11]*
B. Neck
   1. Meaning
      a. Pivotal
      b. Links the head and torso
      c. Houses the spinal cord
      d. Nerves and blood vessels pass through
      e. Holds the head up
      f. Turns head to look, listen, smell, and taste
   2. Applications of massage
      a. Chronic neck tension
      b. Neck stiffness
      c. Tension headache
      d. In treatment for whiplash and torticollis (wry neck)
   3. Review muscular anatomy of neck
      a. Superficial muscles
      b. Deep muscles *[See Figure 10-12]*
      c. Endangerment sites
         a. Anterior neck
         b. Carotid artery and jugular vein
   4. Techniques to integrate into neck massage
      a. Direct pressure to posterior cervical muscles *[See Figure 10-13]*
      b. Deep pressure to suboccipital muscles *[See Figure 10-14]*
      c. Direct pressure to thoracic attachments—supine
      d. Neck massage—prone
         1. Warm posterior cervical muscles with effleurage
         2. One-hand kneading *[See Figure 10-15]*
         3. Direct pressure along posterior cervical muscles
         4. Direct pressure to thoracic attachments
C. Back
   1. Meaning
      a. Core for upright posture

     b. Attachment for arms and legs

     c. Prone to tension, aches, and pains

     d. Poor sitting posture leads to back ache

     e. Holds worry and anxiety (i.e., "weight of the world")

     f. Bent-over posture evokes image of weakness

     g. Standing tall presents image of strength

2. Applications of massage

     a. Soothing back massage—nurturing, sympathy

     b. Deep relaxation

     c. Help with restful sleep

     d. Release tension from physical labor

     e. Relieve tension headache along with neck massage

3. Review muscular anatomy of back

     a. Three-dimensional concept of back—layers of muscles

     b. Sides of torso are part of the back

     c. Shoulder muscles attach on the back

     d. Groups of muscles from upper to lower back

4. Techniques to integrate into back massage

     a. Skin rolling *[See Figure 7-16]*

     b. Warming friction of the back *[See Figures 7-18 and 7-19]*

     c. Effleurage between the ribs *[See Figure 10-16]*

5. Therapeutic sequence for the lower back *[Summary Table 10-1] [See Figures 10-17 and 10-18]*

6. Back massage for relaxation

     a. Avoid specific painful techniques.

     b. Apply long flowing effleurage with oil.

     c. "Seamless" feel to slow continuous strokes

     d. Vary pattern to avoid boredom.

     e. Integrate kneading of shoulders for variety.

     f. Finish with nerve strokes or passive touch over scapulae.

7. Sedating effleurage of the back

     a. To help patients and clients fall asleep

     b. Can be performed without oil or lotion

     c. Technique

        1. Long gliding strokes directly over the spine

        2. Performed from base of skull to coccyx

        3. Alternate hands for continuous feel

        4. Pressure light but firm

        5. Monotonous rhythm

        6. Limit to 2–3 minutes

D. Buttocks

1. Meaning

     a. Support the entire body.

     b. Provide power for locomotion.

     c. Associated with sex appeal.

     d. Source of embarrassment in some.

     e. Source of psychological pain for physically or sexually abused.

2. Applications of massage

     a. Relieve stress from sports and physical activity.

     b. Relieve stiffness from lack of movement.

   c. Relieve sciatic pain from nerve impingement.
   d. Increase mobility at hip joint for improved locomotion.
  3. Review muscular anatomy of the hip.
   a. Superficial muscles—gluteals
   b. Deeper muscles *[See Figure 10-19]*
  4. Techniques to integrate into massage of the buttocks
   a. Use of elbow and forearm *[See Figure 10-20]*
   b. Use of fist *[See Figure 10-21]*
   c. Direct pressure to gluteal attachments
   d. Mobilizations and stretching *[Refer to Chapter 8]*
 E. Lower extremities
  1. Meaning
   a. Principal means of locomotion for human beings.
   b. Afford a great degree of mobility and independence.
   c. Loss of use means greater dependence and loss of freedom.
   d. "Spring in step" is sign of vitality.
   e. Walking and running are important fitness activities.
   f. Shoes are worn for protection but also confine the feet.
   g. If your feet hurt, you hurt all over.
   h. Foot massage is pleasurable treat.
  2. Applications of massage
   a. For people who stand long hours in their jobs
   b. Strained feet from shoes with poor support
   c. For sedentary people
  3. Review of muscular anatomy of lower extremities
   a. Thigh muscles
   b. Iliopsoas *[See Figure 10-22]*
   c. Lower leg muscles
   d. Feet
   e. Endangerment sites (e.g., popliteal area)
   f. Contraindications (e.g., varicose veins, phlebitis, athlete's foot, bunions)
  4. Therapeutic foot massage sequence *[Summary Table 10-2; Figure 10-23]*
  5. Therapeutic sequence for enhancing mobility in the lower extremities *[Summary Table 10-3; Figures 10-24, 10-25, 10-26]*
 F. Upper extremities
  1. Meaning
   a. Human ability to grasp and manipulate objects
   b. Used for activities of daily living
   c. Used for hobbies and sports
   d. Important for communication
   e. Gestures of friendliness and affection
   f. Loss of use of arms can be devastating.
  2. Applications of massage
   a. For preventing and treating repetitive strain injuries
   b. For maintaining shoulder flexibility
   c. To restore lost mobility
  3. Review of muscular anatomy of upper extremities
   a. Shoulders
   b. Upper arm

    c. Forearm

    d. Hands

  4. Therapeutic sequence for enhancing mobility in the shoulder girdle *[Summary Table 10-4; Figures 10-27, 10-28, 10-29]*

  5. Preventing forearm strain

    a. Warm forearms with general massage

    b. Deep thumb stripping to anterior and posterior muscles *[See Figure 10-30]*

    c. Circular friction to muscle attachments at the elbow

    d. Direct pressure to forearm muscle bellies

    e. Mobilizing techniques for the wrist

    f. Stretches for the wrist

    g. General hand massage

    h. Finish with effleurage from hand to shoulder

G. Chest and abdomen

  1. Meaning

    a. Chest

      1. Movement of breathing is evidence of life itself.

      2. Women's breasts associated with nurturing and sex appeal.

      3. Men's chests associated with strength and power.

      4. Drape women's breasts at all times.

      5. Breast massage requires special training and informed consent of recipient to perform.

    b. Abdomen

      1. Vulnerable area that lacks bony protection

      2. Contains visceral organs

      3. "Visceral" means deeply felt, elemental emotions

  2. Applications of massage

    a. Gain and maintain good postural alignment

    b. Condition muscles of respiration

    c. Breast massage

    d. Abdominal massage to enhance digestion and elimination

  3. Review anatomy of front of torso

    a. Chest and breast

    b. Abdomen

  4. Massage for rounded shoulders

    a. Massage along with stretching and strengthening program

    b. Includes relaxing and elongating pectoral muscles and anterior deltoid

      1. Warm up area with massage

      2. Compression over anterior deltoid *[See Figure 10-31]*

      3. Circular friction along sternal and clavicular attachments of pectoralis major

      4. Deep effleurage along length of pectoralis minor

      5. Direct pressure over attachments of pectoralis minor *[See Figure 10-32]*

      6. Overhead stretch *[Refer to Figure 8-8]*

      7. Seated pectoral stretch *[See Figure 10-33]*

  5. Therapeutic sequence for enhancing respiration *[Summary Table 10-5; Figures 10-34, 10-35]*

  6. Abdominal massage *[Refer to Chapter 9]*

SUGGESTED CLASSROOM ACTIVITIES

- Ask students to color in different regions on a body outline, anterior and posterior, and write a few sentences about the meaning of regions to them personally. Discuss differences and similarities between students' drawings and answers. Discuss implications for giving massage.

- After full-body massage, ask students to identify how they felt when different areas of the body were touched. Discuss differences and implications for giving massage.

- Demonstrate massage for each body region to accompany lecture.

- Use anatomical models, videos, and/or computer programs for detailed review of anatomy of different regions to accompany lecture.

- After lecture on massage of a body region, students practice integrating additional techniques into full-body sequence.

- With information from recipient interview and health history, students plan massage sessions to include specific techniques to address individual patient/client needs.

- Students practice therapeutic sequences for lower back, foot massage, enhancing mobility in lower extremities, enhancing mobility in shoulders, enhancing respiration.

11

Hydrotherapy/Thermal Therapies

LECTURE OUTLINE

I. History of Hydrotherapy
   A. Definition of hydrotherapy
   B. Ancient use of water in health and healing
      1. Mineral and hot springs
      2. Mayan sweatbaths
      3. Finnish sauna
      4. Roman and Turkish baths
   C. Water-based therapies
      1. Hippocrates (c. 460 B.C.E.)
      2. Vincent Priessnitz (c. 1840 C.E.)
      3. Sebastian Kneipp (c. 1880 C.E.)
      4. European Spas [*See Figure 11-1 KneippTreatment: Upper Affusion with Hose at the Biltz Sanitarium in Weisbaden, Germany 1898*]
      5. Battle Creek Sanitarium and J. Harvey Kellogg
   D. Hydrotherapy in Medicine
      1. Winternitz of Vienna in nineteenth century
      2. Mineral water hospitals in England in nineteenth century
      3. Doctors of biomedicine versus naturopaths and natural healers
      4. Physical therapy in twentieth century

II. Healing Properties of Water
   A. Different uses of water
   B. Temperature ranges for hydrotherapy [*See Table 11-1 Temperature Sensations for Thermo-, Neutro-, and Cryo-Hydrotherapy; Table 11-2 Temperature Ranges for Hydrotherapy and Thermal Therapy Methods from Cold to Hot Applications*]

III. Hydrotherapy Facilities in Spas and Health Clubs
   A. Benefits of typical hydrotherapy facilities [*See Table 11-3 General Effects of Hydrotherapy Comparing Thermo-Hydrotherapy and Cryo-Hydrotherapy*]
   B. Whirlpool bath
      1. Description
      2. Temperature

      3. Healing effects
      4. Hot tubs
  C. Showers
      1. Description
      2. Cold showers
      3. Swiss shower
      4. Vichy shower
      5. Other
  D. Steam room
      1. Description
      2. Temperature
      3. Healing effects
      4. Steam cabinet
      5. Facial steam
  E. Sauna
      1. Description
      2. Temperature
      3. Use with cold plunge
  F. Contraindications for thermo-hydrotherapy *[See Table 11-4 Contraindications for Thermo-Hydrotherapy]*
  G. Guidelines for safe use of hydrotherapy facilities
      1. Time limits
      2. Recovery from over exposure
      3. General guidelines *[See Table 11-5 Guidelines for Safe Use of Thermo-Hydrotherapy Facilities: Whirlpool, Shower, Steam Room, and Sauna]*

IV. Thermo-Therapy: Hot Applications
  A. General benefits
  B. Cellular effects
  C. Contraindications
      1. Raising core body temperature *[See Table 11-4 Contraindications for Thermo-Hydrotherapy]*
      2. Local contraindications
          a. Burns, wounds, swelling, rashes
          b. Other tissue conditions that might be made worse by use of heat
  D. Hot packs and massage
      1. Benefits of hot packs prior to massage
          a. Muscle relaxation
          b. Enhance local circulation
          c. Prepare area for massage
      2. Benefits of hot packs after massage
          a. Enhance muscle relaxation
          b. Prolong increased local circulation
      3. Types of hot packs
          a. Moist hot packs
          b. Dry hot packs
      4. Use of moist hot packs
          a. Hydrocollator units
          b. Temperature range
          c. Use of towels to protect skin

      d. Importance of client feedback and visual check

      e. Caution with clients taking medication that reduces sensation

      f. General guidelines *[See Table 11-6 Summary of Guidelines for Safe Use of Moist Hot Packs Before and During Massage]*

V. Thermal Therapy: Cold Applications

  A. Effects of cold applied locally

    1. Vasoconstriction and decreased local circulation

    2. Decrease in cell metabolism, nerve conduction velocity, pain, muscle spindle activity, and spasm

    3. Lower core body temperature

    4. After tissue trauma, decreases secondary cell and tissue damage

  B. First aid for trauma from strain, sprain, or blow to soft tissues

    1. Benefits as first aid

      a. Limits hemorrhaging and swelling

      b. Limits secondary cell hypoxia or damage

    2. R.I.C.E.S. (rest, ice, compression, elevation, stabilization)

  C. Typical settings for cryotherapy

    1. Sports settings

    2. Rehabilitation settings

    3. Chiropractic offices

  D. Contraindications to local cold applications *[See Table 11-7 Contraindications for Cryo-Hydrotherapy and Cold Applications]*

  E. Cold packs

    1. Commercial cold packs

    2. Ice packs

    3. Used in conjunction with massage

      a. Reduce muscle spasm

      b. Reduce swelling from recent injury

      c. Reduce pain

      d. Replace massage if massage is contraindicated locally around injury site

      e. General Guidelines *[See Table 11-8 Summary of Guidelines for Safe Use of Cold and Ice Packs Before and During Massage]*

  F. Ice massage

    1. General description

    2. Uses

    3. Ice cups

    4. Technique

      a. Circular motion

      b. Over small area

      c. 5–10 minutes

      d. Until area is numb

    5. Four stages of feeling

      a. Cold

      b. Tingling or itching

      c. Pain, aching, or burning

      d. Numbing

    6. General guidelines for ice massage *[See Table 11-8 Summary of Guidelines for Safe Use of Cold and Ice Packs Before and During Massage]*

SUGGESTED CLASSROOM ACTIVITIES

- Invite a panel of three to five massage practitioners from a variety of settings (e.g., spa, health club, rehabilitation clinic, athletic training department, chiropractic office) to describe the use of hydrotherapy and thermal therapies in their settings. Variation: Invite a single presenter from a setting with special relevance to the students.

- Take a field trip to a spa or health club with good hydrotherapy facilities. Ask the facilities manager to take the class on a tour, talk about how facilities are used by patrons, and about facility maintenance. If possible, arrange for students to experience the hydrotherapy offered at the facility.

- Take a field trip to a rehabilitation or athletic training facility. Ask a therapist or trainer to describe the types of hydrotherapy or thermal therapies available there, and show the relevant facilities and equipment. If possible, arrange for students to observe some applications of hydrotherapy and thermal therapies used.

- Collect a variety of hot packs including moist hot packs, dry hot packs, and other commercial products for the therapeutic application of heat. Have students experience different types of products, and rate them on their perceived effectiveness and ease of use. Include products heated in hydrocollator units, microwave ovens, and other sources of heat.

- Collect a variety of cold and ice packs. Have students experience different types of products, and rate them on their perceived effectiveness and ease of use.

- Have students practice applying ice packs to partners, and experiencing the four stages of feeling as cold is applied. Ask receivers to describe what they are feeling, and givers to write down the descriptions and timing of different stages.

- Assign the writing of theoretical case studies in the use of hydrotherapy or thermal therapy methods in conjunction with massage. The written reports should include a general description of the recipient, the indications or reasons for using the chosen method(s), relevant contraindications, desired outcomes, and description of application. Variation: Actual cases where hydrotherapy or thermal therapies were used in conjunction with massage.

- In massage therapy classes, or student clinic, have students practice using hot packs before and during massage sessions.

- Invite a representative from a company making hydrotherapy equipment to speak to the class and answer questions about their products.

12

Myofascial Massage

LECTURE OUTLINE

I. Overview of Myofascial Massage
   A. Fascial anatomy—fibrous connective tissue that holds the body together and gives it shape
   B. Intent of myofascial massage is to release restrictions in fascial tissues.
   C. Goal of myofascial techniques
      1. Stretch fascial sheets
      2. Break fascial adhesions
      3. Leave fascial tissues more pliable
   D. Result of fascial restrictions
      1. Limited mobility
      2. Postural distortion
      3. Poor cellular nutrition
      4. Pain
      5. Variety of other dysfunctions

II. History
   A. Bindegewebsmassage, Elizabeth Dicke of Germany in 1920s
   B. Rolfing, Ida Rolf in United States in 1970s
   C. *Myofascial release* is a term coined by Robert Ward in 1960s
   D. Myofascial release (MFR), John Barnes in 1980s
   E. Other names for myofascial massage: myofascial release, myofascial unwinding, myofascial manipulation

III. The Nature of Fascia
   A. Loose irregular connective tissue *[See Figure 12-1]*
   B. Function
      1. Support
      2. Protection
      3. Separation
      4. Cellular respiration
      5. Elimination
      6. Metabolism
      7. Fluid flow

8. Immune system function
9. Connects the body as a whole in continuous sheet
C. Three primary elements
1. Gel-like ground substance
2. Collagen
3. Elastin
D. *Thixotropy* is a characteristic of fascia.
1. Can change from a more solid to a more liquid gel consistency
2. Becomes more pliable with movement, stretching, heat
E. Fascial sheets are formed by hydrogen bonds between collagen fibers.
F. Depths of fascial tissues
1. Subcutaneous fascia
2. Deep fascia
3. Subserous fascia
4. Deepest fascia
G. Fascial structures
1. Give the body contour (e.g., body straps, retinaculae)
2. Fascial sheaths surround muscles and link muscle groups *[See Figure 12-2]*
H. Metaphor of the knitted sweater to describe interconnectedness of fascia

IV. Myofascial Techniques
A. Four techniques identified by Reihl
1. Skin rolling
2. Arm and leg pulls, and full body stretches
3. Cross-handed stretches
4. Transverse plane releases (pelvic floor, diaphgram, thoracic)
B. Three techniques described by Scheumann
1. Skin lift and roll
2. Myofascial spread
3. Myofascial mobilization, similar to cross-fiber and circular friction
C. Effective myofascial techniques
1. For freeing subcutaneous fascia—skin lifting and rolling *[See Figure 12-3]*
2. Horizontal stretch of superficial fascia—cross-hand stretches *[See Figures 12-4; 12-5]*
3. Horizontal fingertip stretch of fascial restrictions *[See Figure 12-6]*
4. Horizontal forearm stretch of deeper fascia *[See Figure 12-7]*

V. Guidelines for Myofascial Massage *[Summary Table 12-1]*
1. Use observation of posture, palpation skills, and knowledge of fascial anatomy to identify areas of fascial restriction.
2. Choose myofascial massage techniques suitable for the area, and for the depth at which you are working.
3. Use no or very little lubricant so that you can feel fascial restrictions, and apply techniques without sliding over the skin.
4. Make gentle contact and enter tissues slowly until a point or area of resistance is felt.
5. Shift tissues horizontally once you are at the depth you wish to affect.
   • Avoid compressing tissues into bone.
6. Hold a stretch of fascial tissues until they release, usually in 2-5 minutes.
   • Maintain a continuous stretch.
   • Release feels like "melting," softening or "giving" in tissues.
7. Flow with the tissues. Let the direction of the stretch be determined by which way the tissues seem to want to release.

8. Exit tissues with as much care and awareness as when you melted into them.

9. Let fascial tissues rest and integrate after a stretch.

SUGGESTED CLASSROOM ACTIVITIES

- Show *Tappan's Handbook* CD-ROM Video Myofascial Techniques segment to accompany lecture.

- Show video tape of human cadaver dissection that identifies fascia and fascial anatomy. Variation: Arrange for workshop or class visit to college anatomy laboratory to study fascial anatomy.

- Use actual knitted sweater for demonstration of sweater metaphor for the interconnectedness of fascia in the body.

- Demonstrate myofascial techniques described in the text to accompany lecture. Suggestion: Use video camera and monitors for large groups.

- Lead students through myofascial restriction palpation drills.

  - 1: Students explore horizontal movement of skin on their own hands and arms using their fingertips, noting differences in mobility and elasticity in different areas. Variation: Perform same drill on one or more partners.

  - 2: Recipient is face down on the massage table with back undraped. Students explore for elasticity and adhering using gentle skin lifting technique noting areas where superficial tissues seem to be "stuck" to those underneath. Map out (i.e., draw or shade in) the degree of adhering on a blank chart of the upper body.

  - 3: Repeat 2 after warming the area thoroughly with massage. Note differences in degree of pliability of subcutaneous tissues.

  - Using fingertips for deeper penetration into soft tissues [*See Figure 12-6*], have students explore a partner's back for fascial restrictions by stretching tissues horizontally. Emphasize the subtle nature of the palpation. When they feel a resistance, have them hold the stretch until they feel a "melting" and elongation of tissues.

- Lead students through practice of myofascial techniques mentioned in the chapter.

- Invite a professional massage therapist who specializes in myofascial techniques, or is certified in a specific myofascial approach, to demonstrate his or her work, talk to the class, and answer questions.

13

Neuromuscular Therapy

LECTURE OUTLINE

I. Overview of Neuromuscular Therapy (NMT)
  A. NMT techniques deactivate tender spots in myofascial tissues called trigger points (TrP)
  B. TrPs can result from several factors such as trauma or muscle overload
  C. TrPs cause dysfunction such as pain, weakness, limited flexibility

II. History of Neuromuscular Massage
  A. Stanley Lief had world famous natural healing resort in England in 1925
  B. Janet Travell, M.D. provided TrP treatment to two American presidents in the 1960s, and with D. Simons wrote a definitive work on trigger points.
  C. Bonnie Prudden developed a systematic approach to treating trigger points called *Myotherapy*.
  D. Others have developed systems of trigger point therapy under the general designation of neuromuscular therapy (NMT)

III. Nature of Trigger Points
  A. Characteristics
    1. Small tender spots in muscles that may radiate pain when pressed
    2. Palpated as taut bands of tissue
  B. Defined by Travell as "a focus of hyperirritability in a tissue that, when compressed is:
    1. Locally tender, and is sufficiently hypersensitive
    2. Gives rise to referred pain and tenderness
    3. Sometimes referred to as "autonomic phenomena and distortion of proprioception."
  C. Referral Patterns
    1. Pain referred to TrP's zone of reference
    2. Referred pain described as dull and aching, deep, with intensity varying from low-grade discomfort to severe
    3. Variations
      a. Pain with or without pressure on the spot
      b. Pain at rest or in motion
    4. Signs of trigger points
      a. Pressing point elicits pain in zone of reference.
      b. Involved muscle may be stiff, weak, motion restricted.

      c. Attempts to stretch the muscles elicit pain.

      d. Muscles in immediate area feel tense and ropelike.

    5. Examples of phenomena in zone of reference triggered by active TrPs.

      a. Pain and tenderness

      b. Spasm

      c. Pilomotor response (i.e., goose bumps)

      d. Vasodilation

      e. Increased gland secretion

    6. Common trigger point locations *[Refer to Figure 13-1]*

  D. Varieties of trigger points

    1. *Latent* TrP are only painful when pressed.

    2. *Active* trigger points

      a. Always tender

      b. Prevent full muscle lengthening

      c. Weaken the muscle

      d. Refer pain on direct compression

    3. *Primary* trigger points are activated directly by trauma, overload, etc.

    4. *Secondary* trigger points are reactions from primary TrPs.

    5. *Satellite* trigger points are in zone of reference of a primary TrP.

    6. *Associated* trigger points refer to secondary or satellite TrPs.

  E. Origins of trigger points

    1. Direct

      a. Overload or overwork of muscle

      b. Trauma to a muscle

      c. Chilling of a muscle

    2. Indirect

      a. Arthritic joints

      b. Emotional distress

      c. Certain visceral diseases

      d. Other TrPs (i.e., associated trigger points)

    3. Common activities that cause trigger points

      a. Repetitive tasks (e.g., athletes, musicians, physical laborers)

      b. Poor posture that strains muscles

IV. Locating Trigger points

  A. Client complaints

    1. Muscle tension causing pain and weakness

    2. Muscle shortening causing loss of flexibility

    3. Describe a common TrP referral pattern

  B. Clients map out areas of pain on a blank chart

  C. Palpation

    1. Felt as taut bands in muscles

    2. Ropelike feel to muscles in area

  D. Verbal feedback from client regarding location and severity of TrP

    1. Helps in finding exact location and best angle for direct pressure

    2. Pain reported is often greater than expected for amount of pressure used on the point

    3. "Jump sign" or outcry from client when TrP is pressed

V. Deactivation Techniques

  A. Nonmanual methods (beyond scope of massage therapy)

    1. Spray and stretch

       2. Saline injection
       3. Dry needling
       4. Anesthetics
  B. Manual methods
       1. Ischemic compression with thumb or hand tool
       2. Deep stroking or stripping over the area
       3. Deep friction at TrP site
       4. Vibration
       5. Methods followed by stretch of affected muscles
  C. Ischemic compression techniques
       1. Cause blanching with hypoxia followed by reactive hyperemia
       2. Pressure applied for 20–60 seconds
       3. Tissue compression is gradual and deep enough to engage the TrP
       4. Pressure is released when tension fades or client reports relief
       5. Examples
            1. Thumb pressure *[See Figure 13-2]*
            2. Thumb pressure *[See Figure 13-3]*
            3. Finger pressure *[See Figure 13-4]*
            4. Use of elbow *[See Figure 13-5]*
            5. Use of hand tool *[See Figure 13-6]*
            6. Squeezing technique *[See Figure 13-7]*
       6. Important to finish with stretch to lengthen tissues

SUGGESTED CLASSROOM ACTIVITIES

- Show *Tappan's Handbook* CD-ROM Video Neuromuscular Massage segment.

- Using a blank chart of the body, front and back, students shade in their own areas of muscle tension and location of tender spots.

- In partners, students press spots indicated on TrP charts (above) to feel for taut or ropey bands of tissue. Receivers give feedback about tenderness and referred pain.

- Students compare results of above exercise with standard TrP chart.

- Demonstrate different methods of deactivating TrPs on model.

- Invite a professional massage practitioner specializing in neuromuscular massage, or certified in NMT, to demonstrate their techniques for deactivating TrPs to the class.

- Show instructional video on neuromuscular massage or NMT.

- Students practice locating and deactivating TrPs on practice partners.

- Students practice integrating trigger point deactivation into full-body massage.

14

Lymphatic Drainage Massage

LECTURE OUTLINE

I. Overview of Lymphatic Drainage Massage (LDM)
  A. LDM refers to systems of soft tissue manipulation designed to assist the function of the lymphatic system.
  B. LDM techniques are gentle, slow, repetitive strokes performed in a specific direction and sequence to enhance lymphatic circulation.
  C. Uses of LDM
    1. General wellness
    2. Enhance soft tissue healing; reduce edema
    3. Treat lymphedema

II. History of LDM
  A. Western scientific studies in the late nineteenth century examined the use of massage to increase lymphatic flow.
  B. Alexander von Winiwarter, a German surgeon, treated lymphedema with combination cleanliness, compression, exercise, and massage in 1880s.
  C. Emil and Astid Vodder developed Vodder's Manual Lymph Drainage in 1930s.
  D. Michael and Ethel Foldi developed Complete Decongestive Therapy (CDT) for treating lymphedema in 1970s.
  E. Techniques of lymphatic drainage massage continue to be developed to enhance health, facilitate soft tissue healing, and treat lymphedema.

III. Lymphatic System and LDM
  A. Lymph fluid: water, protein molecules, cellular components, fatty acids
  B. Lymphatic system vessels
    1. Initial lymphatics, aka lymph capillaries *[See Figure 14-1]*
      a. Located in almost all tissues and organs
      b. One cell thick with openings to let in fluid and fatty acids
      c. Flaps prevent backflow of fluid
      d. Traction on anchoring filaments helps open flaps
      e. Heavy pressure closes flaps
    2. Precollector vessels
    3. Collectors

          a. Valved vessels

          b. Lymphangions—contractile smooth muscle segments

    C. Pattern of lymph flow *[See Figure 14-2]*

    D. Lymph nodes

        1. Clusters located in head, neck, chest, abdomen, and groin

        2. Contain macrophages that remove bacteria, cell debris, and foreign material

        3. Superficial drainage pathways leading to nodes *[See Figure 14-3]*

IV. Indications and Contraindications

    A. Indications

        1. Conditions that involve lymphatic blockages: allergies, arthritis, colds, colitis, edema, sinus congestion, psoriasis

        2. Musculoskeletal injuries

        3. Primary lymphedema

        4. Secondary lymphedema caused by surgery, radiation therapy, trauma, tumors, scarring, chronic infections

    B. Contraindications

        1. Infection

        2. Malignant tumors

        3. Thrombosis

        4. Phlebitis

        5. Major heart problems

        6. Any condition potentially worsened by increased fluid circulation (e.g., kidney disease, asthma, thyroid conditions)

V. Lymphatic Drainage Massage

    A. Follows a specific sequence of application and uses techniques specifically designed to improve lymph flow

    B. Five important factors in applying LDM techniques (Reihl)

        1. Correct pressure

          a. Light—about 1–4 ounces of pressure

          b. Only enough to cause superficial traction of skin

        2. Direction

          a. Active part is towards the targeted node

          b. Skin "snaps back" when released

        3. Rhythm

          a. Alternating active and passive phases

          b. Repeated 6–8 times in regular rhythm

        4. Sequence through superficial lymph pathways

        5. Contraindications

    C. Techniques *[Tappan's Handbook CD-ROM Video Lymphatic Drainage Massage Segment]*

        1. Stationary circles *[See Figure 14-4]*

        2. Scoop technique *[See Figure 14-5]*

VI. Basic Principles of LDM

        1. Lymph is pushed toward the nodes in a specific sequence.

        2. The area proximal to a node is treated before the distal area so that the proximal area is emptied to make room for the fluid flowing in from the distal end.

        3. Pressure is limited to just enough to move the skin, about 1–4 ounces.

        4. With each movement the skin is stretched with enough intensity that it "snaps back" when released.

5. There is a rest or zero pressure phase after each stroke to let lymph move through the vessels.
6. The techniques and variations are repeated rhythmically, usually six to eight times, either at the same location in stationary circles or in expanding spirals. The inertial mass of the tissue fluid needs time and repetition before it responds.
7. The pressure phase of a circle lasts longer than the relaxation phase.
8. As a rule, reddening of the skin should *not* appear.
9. Techniques should *not* elicit pain.

VII. Application of LDM
   A. Effect of LDM largely derived from mechanical displacement of lymph fluid and the substances it carries.
   B. LDM techniques require sensitivity and precision.
   C. General rule: The softer the tissue, the softer techniques should be.
   D. Specific application is determined by practitioner's knowledge, skill, experience, intuition.

SUGGESTED CLASSROOM ACTIVITIES

- Show *Tappan's Handbook* CD-ROM Video Segment on Lymphatic Drainage Massage to go along with lecture.

- Demonstrate LDM techniques to illustrate information from lecture.

- Using washable markers or crayons (e.g., china markers) have students locate the lymph nodes on the arms and legs, and trace drainage pathways as shown in Figure 14-3.

- Invite a professional massage practitioner specializing in lymphatic massage, or certified in a specific form of LDM, to demonstrate his or her technique to the class, to describe the sequence and direction of application, and to answer questions.

- Invite to class a massage practitioner trained in a form of LDM and who works with lymphedema patients. Ask him or her to discuss the effects of lymphatic massage techniques on patients, and specific challenges working with this population. Variation: Also invite a lymphedema patient to class to discuss their experience with massage.

- Invite to class a massage practitioner who performs lymphatic massage of the head and neck as a health spa service. Ask him or her to demonstrate the technique, and discuss benefits for general health and beauty. Variation: Invite him or her to instruct the class and lead practice of the spa session.

- Lead students through practice of LDM techniques. Variation: Invite an LDM specialist to instruct the class and lead practice.

- Show an instructional video on lymphatic drainage massage to reinforce lecture.

15

Foot Reflexology

LECTURE OUTLINE

I. Overview
   A. Theory: Pressure applied to specific spots on the feet stimulates corresponding areas in other parts of the body.
   B. Reflexology charts are maps of the feet that help identify which part of body is stimulated when a specific spot of the foot is pressed.
   C. Practitioners integrate foot reflexology into general massage sessions, as well as into foot massage and reflexology sessions.

II. History
   A. Massaging and pressing the feet is an ancient health practice.
   B. Zone Therapy provided the theoretical basis for modern reflexology.
      1. Popularized by William Fitzgerald in early 1900s
      2. Fitzgerald was a respected doctor in Hartford, Connecticut.
      3. Theory showing longitudinal zones from head to toe *[Refer to Figure 15-2]*
   C. Modern foot reflexology can be traced to Eunice Ingham (1889–1974)
      1. Combined Zone Therapy with compression massage of the feet
      2. Physiotherapist and natural healer who developed reflexology in the United States in the 1930–1940s
      3. Created foot charts showing spots on the feet and corresponding body areas *[Refer to Figure 15-1]*
      4. Traveled throughout the United States teaching reflexology in the 1950–1960s
   D. Reflexology is now practiced all over the world.

III. Theories of Reflexology
   A. Zone Therapy—body divided into 10 longitudinal zones with endpoints in the feet *[Refer to Figure 15-2]*
      1. Pressure applied anywhere in the zone affects the entire zone.
      2. Feet are especially sensitive and easily accessed for Zone Therapy.
   B. Eunice Ingham believed that reflexology techniques dissolved crystalline deposits in the feet that interfere with nerve and blood supply.
   C. Kunz and Kunz: reflexology techniques restore "lost balance," and cause relaxation and improved circulation.
   D. Some believe that zones are like energy meridians in Chinese medicine.

IV. Positioning the Receiver
   A. Options for positioning
      1. Lying supine on a massage table
      2. Semireclining on a massage table
      3. Sitting in recliner chair
   B. Use bolster under knees to prevent hyperextension

V. Practitioner Body Mechanics
   A. Maintain good head, neck, and back alignment.
   B. Adjustments for good body mechanics
      1. Adjust table height.
      2. Place bolster under recipient's legs to bring them to proper height.
      3. Adjust the height of the practitioner's chair or stool.
      4. Review good sitting mechanics. *[Refer to Figure 6-21a-b]*

VI. Foot Reflexology Techniques
   A. Thumb walking *[See Figure 15-3]*
   B. Finger walking *[See Figure 15-4]*
   C. Hook and backup *[See Figure 15-5]*
   D. Direct pressure with fingertips *[See Figure 15-6]*
   D. Squeezing *[See Figure 15-7]*

SUGGESTED CLASSROOM ACTIVITIES

- Show the *Tappan's Handbook* CD-ROM Video Reflexology segment to accompany lecture.

- Show an instructional video on reflexology to accompany lecture.

- Present research studies on the effectiveness of reflexology.

- Draw the reflexology chart on a partner's feet using washable markers.

- Demonstrate foot reflexology techniques to accompany lecture.

- Students practice foot reflexology techniques on a partner.

- Invite an experienced and certified reflexologist to demonstrate his or her technique and answer questions from the class.

16

Polarity Therapy

LECTURE OUTLINE

I. Overview
  A. The purpose of polarity therapy techniques is to release obstructions to the free flow of energy through the body to support health and healing.
  B. Polarity techniques involve simple touching and gentle movements such as rhythmic pressing and rocking.
  C. Comprehensive approach to polarity therapy also involves exercises, nutrition and love.

II. History and Philosophy
  A. Polarity therapy was developed by Randolph Stone (1890–1981) in mid-1900s.
    1. Stone was a natural healer trained in chiropractic, naturopathy, and osteopathy.
    2. Stone studied Chinese acupuncture, herbal medicine, Hermetic Kabalistic systems, and Ayurvedic medicine of India.
    3. Fundamental beliefs
      a. Existence of a subtle form of energy that permeates the body and gives it health
      b. Disease is a result of the obstruction of the flow of energy.
      c. Natural healing techniques are effective because they support the individual's innate healing capacity and balance the flow of energy.
    4. Stone synthesized various approaches to natural healing, and relying heavily on Ayurvedic theory, developed polarity therapy.
  B. Pierre Pannetier helped spread the practice of polarity therapy beginning in 1973 after Stone's retirement.
  C. Different schools of polarity therapy have evolved over the years.
    1. Some emphasize the esoteric theory of polarity therapy.
    2. Some emphasize reliance on working intuitively and with direct experience of subtle energies.

III. Physiological Effects
  A. Subjective indications of effects of polarity therapy
    1. Health is often equated with energy.
    2. Polarity therapists feel definite tingling in their hands that varies with the health of the area being treated.
    3. Giver and receiver often feel simultaneous changes in their sense of energy.

B. Objective changes that occur with polarity therapy
  1. Techniques stimulate the body's reflexes.
  2. Rocking techniques induce relaxation, lower muscle tension, reduce pain.
  3. Stimulating joints lowers muscle tone, increases circulation, stimulates endorphin release.
  4. Some rhythmic techniques induce a light hypnotic state, relaxation, and moments of peace.

IV. Principles of Polarity Therapy
  A. Energy
    1. Rubbing palms together exercise to increase energy awareness
    2. Partner exercise "plugging into" each other *[See Figure 16-1]*
  B. Love
    1. *Not* sloppy sentimentality or overbearing affection
    2. It is caring so powerful that it carries with it no agenda, no end result that must be obtained.
    3. Attitude of surrender and openness, getting out of the way of the body's healing tendency
    4. Exercise in quality of love *[See Figure 16-1]*
  C. Removing obstructions
    1. An obstruction is an area of the body where there seems to be a stagnation or holding pattern that interferes with the free flow of energy.
    2. Some obstructions can be assessed visually as poor posture.
    3. Exercise for locating and freeing obstructions *[See Figure 16-2]*
  D. Understanding
    1. Invites the practitioner to be open to the recipient's experience
    2. Pannetier promoted a commonsense approach emphasizing a caring attitude, acceptance, and trust that whatever happens is from clearing energy blocks and is for the best.
    3. Polarity therapy is a gentle art and nothing is ever forced.
    4. Pannetier taught that the giver is not there to rescue the receiver but to plant the seeds of letting go and trusting.
  E. Nutrition and exercise
    1. Exercises suggested include stretching and toning.
    2. Sounds are sometimes used to stimulate energy.
    3. Emphasis is eating in a relaxed state of mind rather than on the particulars of what is eaten.
      a. Dietary suggestions are based on Ayruvedic theory
      b. Sometimes includes cleansing period

V. Basic Polarity Movements
  A. Typically performed in 15–22 movement sessions to balance the entire body
  B. Abbreviated general session
    1. The tenth cranial (cradle) *[See Figures 16-3; 16-4]*
    2. Neck stretch *[See Figure 16-5]*
    3. Tummy rock *[See Figure 16-6]*
    4. Leg pull
    5. Inside ankle press *[See Figure 16-7]*
    6. Outside ankle press *[See Figure 16-8]*
    7. Pelvis and knee rock *[See Figure 16-9]*
    8. Arm-shoulder rotations *[See Figure 16-10]*
    9. Thumb web-forearm stimulation *[See Figure 16-11]*

10. Elbow milk-abdomen rock *[See Figure 16-12]*
11. Pelvic rock *[See Figure 16-13]*
12. Occipital press *[See Figure 16-14]*
13. Cranial polarization *[See Figure 16-15]*
14. Navel-third eye
15. Brushing off to finish *[See Figure 16-16; 16-17]*

SUGGESTED CLASSROOM ACTIVITIES

- Show *Tappan's Handbook* CD-ROM Video Polarity Therapy Segment to accompany lecture.
- Show instructional video on polarity therapy, and discuss similarities and differences in techniques demonstrated and theory presented.
- Invite a practitioner certified by the American Polarity Therapy Association to class to demonstrate a polarity session and discuss the theory they are applying.
- Lead student through the energy awareness exercise described in the chapter (i.e., rubbing palms together and feeling the energy by self and with a partner).
- Lead students through the energy assessment partner exercise shown in Figure 16-1.
- Lead students through the abbreviated polarity therapy session described in Chapter 14 Figures 16-3 to 16-17.

17

Asian Bodywork Therapy Theory

LECTURE OUTLINE

I. Overview
   A. Asian bodywork therapy (ABT) is a term used to describe forms of bodywork with roots in Chinese Medicine.
   B. Several distinct forms of ABT have evolved over the years in countries like China, Japan, and Korea, and have more recently come to North America and Europe. *[See Figure 17-2]*
   C. The scope of practice of ABT includes assessment and treatment of energetic imbalances according to Chinese medicine theory.
   D. ABT techniques include
      1. Touching, pressing or holding meridians and acupoints
      2. Stretching
      3. External application of medicinal plants
      4. Application of heat or cold
      5. Dietary and exercise suggestions
   E. The National Certification Commission for Acupuncture and Oriental Medicine (NCCAOM) certifies ABT practitioners.

II. History
   A. ABT developed from ancient Chinese folk remedies and thousands of years of empirical evidence.
   B. Early writings and philosophies
      1. Earliest known text on Chinese medicine is the Huang Di Nei Jing, the *Yellow Emperor's Classic of Chinese Medicine.*
         a. Thought to have been written in about 2500 B.C.E.
         b. Written as conversation between the emperor and his minister named Qi Bo
      2. Earliest reference to Yin-Yang is in the *Book of Changes* written in about 700 B.C.E.
      3. Naturalist School of philosophy sought to find ways to live in harmony with nature rather than subdue it. Zou Yan (350–270 B.C.E.) was a promoter of this philosophy which influenced development of Chinese medicine.
   C. Foundations of classical Chinese medicine
      1. Concept of Qi or life energy
      2. Channels of energy or meridians

3. Points of contact with Qi called acupoints
  D. Early development
    1. Origins in the barren lands north of the Yellow River in China, where inhabitants used acupuncture, moxibustion, and *anmo* or manual methods to cure various ailments *[See Figure 17-2]*
    2. Over the years Chinese people came to identify the channels and points on the body where their methods produced maximum results, and this led to discovery of the 12 primary and other energy channels. *[See Figure 17-1]*
    3. Early healing practices were influenced by Taoist philosophy, Yin-Yang or Naturalist School of Philosophy
  E. Traditional Asian medicine (TAM) is sometimes used in the West to refer to Chinese medicine. (Also known as traditional Chinese medicine [TCM])
  F. Spread throughout Asia *[See Figure 17-2]*
    1. Chinese medicine spread throughout China and Korea.
    2. Came to Japan as *kampo*, the Chinese way, in about 600 C.E.
    3. Modified according to local beliefs and practices
  G. Spread East to West
    1. Travels of Marco Polo in thirteenth century brought information about China to Europe
    2. French diplomat named Soulie de Morant brought knowledge of acupuncture to Europe and the Americas in 1940s
    3. Immigrants from Asia brought TAM wherever they settled
    4. Namikoshi taught shiatsu at the Palmer School of Chiropractic in Davenport, Iowa from 1953 to 1960.
    5. Great interest in Eastern philosophies and practices during the 1970s when several forms of ABT from Japan were introduced in the United States
      a. DoAnn Kaneko—Anma Shiatsu
      b. Shizuto Masunaga—Zen Shiatsu
      c. Shizuko Yamamoto—Barefoot Shiatsu
      d. Toshiko Phipps—Eclectic Shiatsu
      e. Takashi Nakamura—Amma
    6. Some modern forms developed in West from TAM (e.g., Jin Shin Do®)
  H. West to East
    1. Western medicine was introduced into Japan during the Meiji Restoration (c. 1868) and again after World War II.
    2. Western medicine was adopted in China during the Cultural Revolution of the 1980s.
    3. In many Asian countries today, Western medicine is being integrated with traditional healing practices.

III. Asian and Western Medicine
  A. Western medicine
    1. Cartesian model: split between body and mind
    2. Based on what can be reliably measured, predicted, and controlled
    3. Mechanized view of the body (i.e., body as machine)
    4. Each body system, organ, symptom viewed as separate
    5. Excels at emergency breakdown repair
  B. Traditional Asian Medicine
    1. Universe is dynamic, constantly moving and changing
    2. Humans are natural, integral part of the universe
    3. Humans stand out as waves on the ocean yet are still part of the sea
    4. Humans are related and connected to all that exists

IV. Yin and Yang
   A. Yin/Yang symbol [See Figure 17-3] symbolizes movement and change in the universe
   B. Chinese character for Yin depicts the shady side of the mountain [See Figure 17-3]
      1. Yin is dark, deep, dense aspect of the universe
      2. Yin is feminine, interior, still, substantial, cool, and contracting in contrast to Yang
   C. Chinese character for Yang is a hillside in full sun. [See Figure 17-3]
      1. Yang is light, energetic, ethereal aspects of the universe
      2. Yang is masculine, exterior, moving, nonsubstantial, warm, expanding, and opposing but supporting Yin.
   D. Principles of Yin and Yang
      1. Opposition—Yin and Yang control and restrict each other.
      2. Interdependence—Yin and Yang are relative concepts totally dependent on each other.
      3. Consuming/supporting relationship—Yin and Yang maintain a constant dynamic balance.
      4. Intertransformation—Yin and Yang are constantly transforming into each other.
      5. Infinite divisibility—Everything can be infinitely divided into Yin or Yang
   E. Yin and Yang aspects of the human body
      1. Yin
         a. The front, interior, medial aspects of limbs
         b. Yin organs are those that store the pure essences extracted from food by the Yang organs
      2. Yang
         a. The back, head, exterior, and lateral aspects of limbs
         b. Yang organs transform, digest and excrete food and liquids

V. The Concept of Qi
   A. Big Qi is everything in the universe.
      1. Qi is a continuous form of energy in material form when it condenses and nonmaterial when it disperses.
      2. Chinese character for Qi depicts rice cooking in a pot with steam escaping [See Figure 17-4]
         a. Qi is the rice and the steam, the material and the energy
         b. Qi is matter (e.g., rocks, trees, raindrops) and energy (e.g., sunshine, starlight, movement of the wind)
   B. Little Qi is the life force or life energy (i.e., what makes people go)
      1. Extracted from the food we eat and air we breathe
      2. Transformed into the Qi that circulates through channels (a.k.a. meridians)
      3. TAM aims to harmonize the flow of Qi along with other Fundamental Substances (i.e., Shen, Jing, Blood and Jin/Ye)
         a. If Qi is deficient, one tonifies it.
         b. If Qi is in excess, one disperses it.
         c. If Qi is stagnant, one moves it.
         d. If Qi is sinking, one uplifts it.
         e. If Qi is rebellious, one rectifies it.
   C. Functions of Qi
      1. Transforms
      2. Transports
      3. Holds
      4. Protects
      5. Warms

VI. Five Elements *[See Table 17-1]*
  A. A poetic but scientific way of using natural phenomenon to explore and treat our psyche, spiritual state, anatomy, physiology, and the dynamics of the disease process.
  B. Circle of life is envisioned as the Five Elements.
  C. The Five Elements
    1. Wood
      a. A Yang element
      b. Most evident in spring and at sunrise
      c. Associated with green, wind, sour taste, tears, sight
      d. Power of Wood: to see clearly into the future, plan
      e. Balanced Wood: benevolence, discernment, patience
      f. Unbalanced Wood: belligerent, timid, rigid, indecisive
      g. Expressed in two organs and channels
        1. Liver (Yin)
        2. Gall Bladder (Yang)
    2. Fire
      a. Most Yang element
      b. Most evident in summer and in the heat of the day
      c. Associated with heat, light, sweat, the tongue, the vessels
      d. Ability to feel warm physically and emotionally
      e. Capacity to be loving, passionate, joyful, confident
      f. Balanced Fire: propriety, insight, intimacy
      g. Imbalanced Fire: guardedness, vulnerability, excessive control, apathy
      h. Expressed in four channels
        1. Heart (Yin): governs blood and blood vessels
        2. Small Intestine (Yang): separates pure from impure
        3. Pericardium (Yin): assists heart function
        4. Triple Burner (Yang): regulates digestion, assimilation, elimination
    3. Earth
      a. A Yin element
      b. Most evident in late summer
      c. Felt as change between all of the seasons, transformative quality
      d. Balanced Earth: integrity, altruism, adaptability
      e. Imbalanced Earth: selfishness, martyrs, self-sufficient or needy, stubborn or compliant
      f. Expressed in two channels and organs
        1. Spleen
        2. Stomach
    4. Metal
      a. A Yin element
      b. Most evident in autumn, and felt at dusk
      c. Associated with letting go, grief, rank smell, dry climate, mucus, pungent taste
      d. Balanced Metal: inspired, balanced, receptive
      e. Unbalanced Metal: vanity, self-deprecation, zealotry, despondency
      f. Expressed in two channels
        1. Lung channel
        2. Large intestine channel
    5. Water
      a. The most Yin element
      b. Most evident in winter, at night, in northern direction
      c. Associated with yielding, hearing, fear, sound of groaning, rotten smell, salty taste

       d. Influenced by Water: bones, ears, kidneys, bladder

       e. Balanced Water: wisdom, concentration, contemplation

       f. Imbalanced Water: extremely reckless, scattered, conservative, physically or emotionally dormant

       g. Expressed in two channels

          1. Kidney

          2. Bladder

D. Sheng and Ko Cycles

  1. Sheng Cycle

     a. The creation, generating or promoting cycle

     b. Each element supports the next

     c. Example: Wood feeds the Fire, which creates ash, which becomes Earth

  2. Ko Cycle

     a. The controlling or acting cycle

     b. Each element controls and is in turn controlled by another element

     c. Example: Earth and dam or control Water; Water extinguishes Fire

  3. The Ko Cycle balances the Sheng Cycle to avoid unrestrained growth.

  4. The balanced cyclical relationship of the Five Elements maintaining one another is considered to foster the healthiest life.

E. The Primary Channels and the Chinese Body Clock

  1. Primary Channels (see inside back cover of *Tappan's Handbook*)

     a. Every part of the body, inside and out is enlivened, nourished and warmed by Qi and blood through this network, allowing the body to function as a single unit rather than separate parts.

     b. In addition to the 12 primary channels typically shown in merdian charts there are also 8 extraordinary vessels, 16 luo collaterals, 12 cutaneous regions, minute collaterals, and 12 senew and 12 divergent channels.

     c. The name of each channel has three parts:

        1. The limb (i.e., foot or hand) where it starts

        2. Its six channel relationship with another of the same type (yin or yang)

        3. The organ it relates to (e.g., liver or small intestine)

     d. Charts only show external energy pathways, but the pathways also go to the interior of the body.

  2. Chinese Body Clock Overview *[See Table 17-2]*

     a. Channels flow through the body according to a natural, rhythmic cycle

     b. Each channel has its peak flow when its Qi is at its maximum

     c. Each channel has its weak flow when its Qi is at its minimum

  3. Times and Channels in the Chinese Body Clock

     a. 3:00–5:00 A.M. Hand Taiyin Lung Channel

        1. Humans awaken, stretch, and breathe deeply

        2. Relates to Metal Element

        3. Trace path of the Lung Channel

     b. 5:00–7:00 A.M. Hand Yangming Large Intestine Channel

        1. Bowel movement, letting go of the unnecessary

        2. Relates to Metal Element

        3. Trace path of the Large Intestine Channel

     c. 7:00–9:00 A.M. Foot Yangming Stomach Channel

        1. Breakfast, aiding digestion

        2. Relates to Earth Element

        3. Trace path of the Stomach Channel

d. 9:00–11:00 A.M. Foot Taiyin Spleen Channel
   1. Workday begins, accomplishments
   2. Relates to Earth Element
   3. Trace path of the Spleen Channel
e. 11:00 A.M.–1:00 P.M. Hand Shaoyin Heart Channel
   1. Heart of the day, energy strongest
   2. Relates to the Fire Element
   3. Trace path of the Heart Channel
f. 1:00–3:00 P.M. Hand Taiyang Small Intestine Channel
   1. Might get aching shoulders
   2. Related to Fire Element
   3. Trace path of the Small Intestine Channel
g. 3:00–5:00 P.M. Foot Taiyang Bladder Channel
   1. Energy is strongest
   2. Related to Water Element
   3. Trace path of the Bladder Channel
h. 5:00–7:00 P.M. Foot Shaoyin Kidney Channel
   1. Deficient Kidney Qi leads to fatigue
   2. Related to Water Element
   3. Trace path of Kidney Element
i. 7:00–9:00 P.M. Hand Jueyin Pericardium Channel
   1. Time to curl up or hug someone
   2. Related to Fire Element
   3. Trace path of Pericardium Element
j. 9:00–11:00 P.M. Hand Shaoyang Triple Burner Channel
   1. Warm yourself up by rubbing upper arm
   2. Related to Fire Element
   3. Trace path of Triple Burner Channel
k. 11:00pm–1:00 A.M. Foot Shaoyang Gall Bladder Channel
   1. The time when if you can't decide, you "sleep on it"
   2. Related to the Wood Element
   3. Trace convoluted path of the Gall Bladder Channel
l. 1:00–3:00 A.M. Foot Jueyin Liver Channel
   1. Finishes the cycle
   2. Related to Wood Element
   3. Trace path of the Liver Channel
4. Use of Chinese Body Clock as assessment tool
   a. The 24-hour cycle repeats every day
   b. When a problem occurs at a certain time of the day, a look at the related channel could provide clues to the energetic origin of the problem
   c. Might be used to determine the best time for treatment of the channel

VII. Four Pillars of Assessment [See Figure 17-5]
   A. Looking
      1. Physical appearance, demeanor, movement, hair, face color
      2. Color, shape, and coating of the tongue
   B. Touching
      1. Palpate to assess rigidity or flaccidness
      2. Pulse to detect flow of energy through channels

C. Listening and smelling
    1. Listening to the sound quality of the voice
    2. Smelling related to one of the Five Elements (e.g., Earth—fragrant)
D. Asking
    1. About psycho-spiritual-physical functioning
    2. About appetite, diet, digestion, elimination
    3. About sleep patterns, dreaming, relationships, feeling hot or cold, energy levels, menstrual cycle in women
    4. About possible contraindications
E. Also Hara Diagnosis

VIII. Acupoints
A. 365 classical pressure or acupoints located on major energy channels
B. Places where Qi can collect and can be influenced by applying pressure
C. Used for diagnosis as well as treatment of energy imbalances
D. Identified by channel name and point number (e.g., GB20).
E. Effective use based on accurate TAM energy assessment
F. TAM strength is wellness and prevention
G. Points are chosen for the individual's unique situation
H. Twenty useful acupoints [See Table 17-3]
    1. Useful acupoints on the head [See Figure 17-6]
    2. Useful acupoints on the upper body [See Figure 17-7]
    3. Useful acupoints on the arm and shoulder [See Figure 17-8]
    4. Useful acupoints on the leg and hip [See Figure 17-9]
    5. Useful acupoints on the lower leg [See Figure 17-10]

IX. Application of ABT Practice
A. Different forms of Asian bodywork use TAM theory differently, emphasizing different aspects
B. Commonality that binds all ABT forms is the rich history, eloquent theories, and years of development.

SUGGESTED CLASSROOM ACTIVITIES

- Students draw major energy channels on blank outlines of the human body from the front, back and sides. Use different colors for each channel.

- Students trace major energy channels on a partner lying on a massage table. Variation: Draw channels on a partner with washable markers or pencils.

- Students locate the useful acupoints on a partner lying on a massage table. Variation: Draw acupoints on a partner with washable markers or pencils.

- For the above exercises, students compare their finished drawings to a three-dimensional model of Chinese energy channels.

- Invite a certified ABT practitioner to class to demonstrate their ABT form, and explain the theory. Variation: Invite 2–3 ABT practitioners of different forms for comparison.

- Invite a doctor of Chinese medicine to class to demonstrate a TAM diagnosis.

18

Amma: Traditional Japanese Massage

LECTURE OUTLINE

I. Overview
   A. Two Chinese characters pronounced *anmo* (amma in Japanese) mean "to calm by rubbing."
   B. Traditional amma is the foundation of all forms of Japanese acupressure, including modern-day forms of shiatsu.

II. History
   A. Amma has its origins in traditional Chinese medicine, developed in the lands north of the Yellow River thousands of years ago.
      1. Based on a system of meridians and acupressure points called *tsubos,* which make up the energetic anatomy of Chinese medicine.
      2. Anmo was brought to Japan along with other aspects of Chinese culture in the sixth century C.E.
   B. From 600–1600 C.E. amma developed into a highly specialized form of massage involving complex techniques, including a variety of pressing, stroking, stretching, and percussive manipulations.
   C. In the Edo Period of Japanese history (1603–1857 C.E.), medical students studied amma to understand the energetic anatomy of the body, and to learn to administer herbs, and to locate tsubo for acupuncture.
   D. Two events led to the discredit of amma by the Japanese people.
      1. The decree that blind people assume the jobs of amma and acupuncture practitioners as a welfare measure (early 1800s).
      2. During the Meiji Restoration (1868 C.E.) Western medicine began to influence Japanese medical practices.
   E By the beginning of the 1900s, Chinese medicine had become regarded as folk medicine and amma was used primarily for pleasure and comfort. Amma became known as a blind person's profession.
   F. The practice of traditional Japanese arts including amma were outlawed temporarily after World War II.
   G. Shiatsu was created by Torujiro Namikoshi who opened the Japan Shiatsu School in Tokyo in 1940.
      1. Shiatsu incorporates aspects of amma and Western anatomy.

2. Shiatsu was recognized by the Japanese government as a style of massage separate from amma in 1964.
H. Amma in the United States
   1. Torujiro Namikoshi and his son, Toru, brought shiatsu to the United States in the 1950s, teaching it at the Palmer School of Chiropractic in Davenport, Iowa.
   2. In the 1970s a number of practitioners brought their styles of shiatsu to the United States.
      a. DoAnn Kaneko—Anma Shiatsu
      b. Shizuto Masunaga—Zen Shiatsu
      c. Shizuko Yamamoto—Barefoot Shiatsu
      d. Toshiko Phipps—Eclectic Shiatsu
   3. Traditional amma was brought to the United States in 1971 with the opening of Kabuki Hot Springs in Japantown, San Francisco.
      a. Takashi Nakamura from the Kensai School of Massage in Osaka, Japan came to San Francisco in 1977 to teach a amma routine for Kabuki Hot Springs.
      b. A one-hour choreographed amma massage was developed for patrons of the spa including 25 different amma techniques to stimulate over 140 tsubo.
   4. A chair massage routine based on amma was created by David Palmer in the 1980s, who also developed the first special massage chair to bring amma massage to the public's attention.

III. One-Hour Amma Form
  A. General description
   1. Designed as a wellness or health maintenance massage
      a. Relax and rejuvenate
      b. Facilitate energy flow
      c. Improve circulation
   2. Performed with recipient on a massage table
   3. Uses amma techniques: pressing, stroking, stretching, percussion
   4. Stimulates over 140 acupressure points along the 14 major meridians
   5. Rhythmic application in four-beat rhythm
   6. Prescribed sequence called a *kata*
  B. Screening Process
   1. Five basic questions
      a. Have you ever had massage before?
      b. Have you ever had a Japanese massage before?
      c. Have you had any recent injuries or illness?
      d. Are you under a doctor's care or are you taking medication? And to women of child-bearing age:
      e. Are you pregnant or trying to be pregnant?
   2. This amma routine is contraindicated for pregnant women.
   3. Basic approach to contraindications:
      a. When in doubt, don't.
      b. Always error on the side of caution.
   4. Give the receiver instructions to give feedback and choice about the amount of pressure used.
  C. The amma kata
   1. Setup
      a. Receiver is draped with a sheet, and techniques are performed through the sheet. Variation: The receiver is clothed.
      b. Receiver starts face down on the table.

2. Techniques and body sequence
    a. Sequence starts with applying pressure to the back with palms. *[See Figure 18-1]*
    b. Shoulder, arms, hands
    c. Neck, back, hips, legs, feet
        1. Pressing tsubos and along meridians
        2. Finish with percussion
    d. Turn over
    e. Right, then left leg
        1. Pressing tsubos along the leg
        2. Stretching the leg and toes
    f. Face, neck, chest, abdomen
    g. Receiver sits up, and massage scalp, neck, shoulders
    h. Stretch the back and arms
    i. Finish with percussion
    j. End session saying "thank you very much"
        1. Signals that the massage is over
        2. Appreciation for the receiver's cooperation
        3. Practice humility

IV. Amma Techniques
  A. Four basic principles of good body mechanics *[See Tappan's Handbook CD-ROM Video Segment on Asian Bodywork Techniques.]*
    1. Weight transfer
    2. Perpendicularity
    3. Stacking the joints
    4. Keeping the back in alignment
  B. Exercise for practice of principles of good body mechanics *[See Figure 18-2]*
  C. Amma techniques in one-hour sequence *[See Table 18-1]*
    1. Shusho appakuho *[See Figure 18-1]*
    2. Boshi apahuko *[See Figure 18-3]*
    3. Wansho junenko *[See Figure 18-4]*

V. Significance of Using Kata to Teach Massage
  A. *Kata* means "form, sequence, or system of movement that determines precisely how something is accomplished."
  B. Katas are studied in many Japanese arts (e.g., karate, kyudo [zen archery], tea ceremony).
  C. Students practice katas over and over until they become automatic.
  D. Benefits of learning through kata:
    1. Allows practice of skilled touch with confidence.
    2. Kata as developed by a master is proven effective.
    3. Provides practice of point locations.
    4. Student doesn't have to know Chinese medicine; the *kata* knows it.
        a. "The kata is like a wise elder which has the wisdom of the centuries behind it."
        b. "We teach a kata and it is the kata that teaches the student massage."

SUGGESTED CLASSROOM ACTIVITIES

- Show the *Tappan's Handbook* CD-ROM Video segment on Asian bodywork techniques to accompany lecture about good body mechanics.

- Show instructional video about amma to accompany lecture.

- Lead students through the body mechanics exercise described in the chapter *[See Figure 16-2]* and shown in the CD-ROM video. Variation: Apply techniques with client on a massage table and then a massage chair.

- Lead students through practice of amma techniques, and teach a short amma kata.

- Invite an amma practitioner to class to demonstrate amma and explain the techniques and theory.

- Invite a student of a Japanese art that uses the concept of *kata* for learning to demonstrate their kata and explain its purpose. Examples: martial art like karate, kyudo (Zen archery), tea ceremony.

19

Zen Shiatsu: An Overview

LECTURE OUTLINE

I. Introduction to Zen Shiatsu
  A. Zen Shiatsu is a form of Asian bodywork therapy developed by Shizuto Masunaga in Japan and brought to the United States and the West in the 1970s.
  B. Zen Shiatsu is distinguished as having a broader set of meridians and tsubo and uses lighter pressure than other types of shiatsu.

II. History of Shiatsu
  A. In Japan, the use of the hands as a therapeutic tool has a time-honored history and a deep philosophical foundation.
    1. Shi = finger and atsu = pressure in Japanese
    2. Healing with hands has a history in Asia since c. 2500 B.C.E.
  B. Shiatsu is derived from Chinese acupuncture and traditional Japanese massage called amma.
    1. Amma was considered a valuable healing art in Japan until the 1800s.
    2. At that time it was reduced to instrument of pleasure only.
    3. Amma was an occupation for the blind in Japan starting in the late 1800s.
  C. The Nippon Shiatsu School was established in Tokyo by Torujiro Namikoshi in the 1940s.
  D. After the 1940s several styles or forms of shiatsu were developed in Japan, with Zen Shiatsu being created by Shizuto Masunaga.

III. Three major types of Shiatsu have evolved over the years, each of which approaches the goal of balancing energy flow differently.
  A. *Shiatsu massage* as developed by Torujiro Namikoshi and his son Toru.
    1. Based largely on traditional amma techniques
    2. Views body from anatomical and physiological perspective
    3. Pressure is applied to acupoints to relieve symptoms
  B. *Acupressure* is similar to shiatsu massage but incorporates traditional Chinese meridians and tsubos.
  C. *Zen shiatsu* developed by Shizuto Masunaga
    1. Broader set of meridians and tsubos
    2. Lighter pressure
    3. Diagnostic theory of kyo and jitsu

IV. Concepts of Ki and Meridians
  A. Development of theory of energy meridians

1. System of energy meridians was described in the Yellow Emperor's Classic of Internal Medicine written in c. 2500 B.C.E.
2. In China before dissection of the human body was used to study human anatomy, medical theory was based on observation and intuition.
3. Chinese conceptualized the body as a living, dynamic entity subject to the influences of an underlying network of energy pathways.
   B. Emphasis on energy rather than structural anatomy is perhaps the basic difference between Eastern and Western medicine.
   C. Ki (aka *chi* and *qi*) is the life force always present and active within the body.
   1. Common link among all the body's tissues and organs
   2. Keeps organs functional and properly interrelated
   3. Represents the essence of life itself
   4. Affects and controls a person's entire life structure
   D. The unobstructed, balanced flow of ki along the meridians is both the cause and effect of good health.

V. The Structure of Meridians *[See Figure 19-1]*
   A. Each of the meridians has been assigned the name of an organ.
   1. Relationship to the organ is metaphorical rather than physiological. *[Refer to Table 19-1]*
   2. Name refers to the functional influence of the meridian within the body.
   B. Life cycle of meridians
   1. Extracting ki from the environment
      a. Begins with lung and large intestine meridians
      1. Together govern the intake and elimination of ki
      2. The functions of taking in nourishment and eliminating waste must be maintained for good health.
      b. Stomach and spleen meridians
      1. Initiate the intake of food and its breakdown in digestion
      2. Associated with the anatomical stomach, esophagus, duodenum, and digestive enzymes
      c. Heart and small intestine meridians
      1. Nourishment of the psyche by giving meaning to actions
      2. Heart and small intestine meridians most associated with the spiritual aspect of ki, primarily compassion
      3. They are connecting links between the physical and heavenly
      4. Said to influence the quality of the blood
   2. Processing ki internally so that it can be utilized
      a. Bladder and kidney meridians
      1. Filter ki and move it into meridians for circulation
      2. Govern purification and movement process via urination, autonomic nervous system, and endocrine gland system.
      b. Heart constrictor and triple heater meridians
      1. Central distributors of ki
      2. Govern the vascular system, lymphatic system, metabolic processes that regulate temperature
      c. Liver and gall bladder meridians
      1. Control how ki is distributed to accomplish a specific action
      2. Also govern the reproductive system
   C. The meaning of meridian functions can be interpreted on physical, emotional, intellectual, and spiritual levels.

VI. Flow and Quality of Ki
  A. Homeostasis
    1. Dynamic systems naturally seek to maintain overall balance.
    2. Whenever an external force is applied to the system, a change must occur in the system to establish a new order of balance.
    3. Physical, mental, emotional, spiritual stresses (i.e., external forces) produce internal obstructions that upset the balance of ki.
    4. Zen Shiatsu aims to bring the ki back into balance to maintain homeostasis.
  B. Vibrational quality
    1. Ki is a form of vibration that ranges from high to low.
      a. Low vibrational quality seems heavy, slow, cold.
      b. High vibrational quality seems light, fast, heat.
    2. Quantity of ki
      a. Deficient
      b. Excessive
    3. Experienced Zen Shiatsu practitioners develop sensitivity to ki and can sense flow and quality of ki imbalances associated with illness, disease, and pain.
  C. Kyo-Jitsu
    1. Refer to quality and quantity of ki.
    2. Kyo
      a. Area of deficient and weak ki
      b. Absence of ki that retards a meridian's function
    3. Jitsu
      a. Area of excessively strong ki
      b. Usually balances an area of kyo or weakness
    4. Imbalances generally stem from an area of kyo or weakness that leads to areas of jitsu or excess in attempt to compensate for kyo.
    5. Aim of Zen shiatsu is alleviate the area of weakness or kyo to bring the entire system back into balance.

VII. Role of Zen Shiatsu Practitioner
  A. Three primary goals
    1. Diagnosis —To identify the nature and extent of energy balances
    2. Treatment—To penetrate meridians (via tsubos) to balance energy in meridians
    3. Maintenance—To sustain and strengthen energy balance
  B. Diagnosis
    1. To identify the cause and effect relationship between a kyo meridian and a jitsu meridian
    2. Hara diagnosis
      a. Evaluate a person's energy by palpating the abdomen.
      b. Identify meridians out of balance.
      c. Diagnostic areas in abdomen [See Figure 19-2]
      d. Diagnostic areas on back [See Figure19-3]
    3. Hara palpation performed before and after applying techniques (i.e., applying pressure to tsubos).
    4. Final palpation should indicate that both kyo and jitsu conditions have been altered to a state of balance.
  C. Four primary principles of performing shiatsu techniques [See Tappan's Handbook CD-Rom Video Segment on Body Mechanics of Asian Bodywork]
    1. Giver maintains attitude of observer.
      a. Practitioner uses observation to attune to the dynamics of ki in the receiver.
      b. Maintain a relaxed hand and attitude devoid of intent to interfere with receiver's ki.

    c. Receiver's own energy is source of healing; practitioner is simply a catalyst.

  2. Penetration is perpendicular to surface of the meridian.

    a. Energy vortices on meridians are called tsubos (also acupoints).

    b. *Tsubo* means "vase" in Japanese.

    c. Penetration of tsibos must be at 90 degree angle to the tsubo to have maximum effect.

    d. Metaphor of pouring water into a vase without spilling water.

  3. Body weight, leaning into the tsubo, is used to apply pressure

    a. Practitioner's hand and upper body remain relaxed.

    b. Pressure is applied by transferring weight into the hand.

    c. This type of pressure is firm but gentle.

    d. Provides better communication between giver and receiver.

  4. Pressure is applied rhythmically.

    a. Slow rhythm as pressure on tsubo is held for a time.

      1. Used when working along a kyo meridian

      2. Brings the cause of the imbalance to receiver's attention

      3. Allows the receiver's energy time to tune into the area of weakness nd remedy it

      4. Slow rhythm relaxes and soothes

    b. Faster rhythm

      1. Used primarily on jitsu meridians

      2. Causes the ki in tsubos to disperse

      3. Distracts receiver's attention from cause of imbalance

VIII. Shiatsu Perspective

  A. In Chinese medicine, a therapeutic approach was considered valid if it produced consistently positive results over a long period of time with no ill effect.

  B. After thousands of years, shiatsu continues to unify body, mind, and spirit and contributes to a life lived to its highest potential through healthful and fulfilling experiences.

SUGGESTED CLASSROOM ACTIVITIES

- Compare Zen Shiatsu meridian chart (Figure 19-1) to standard Chinese medicine meridian chart on inside back cover of *Tappan's Handbook*.

- Students trace meridians used in Zen Shiatsu on partner's lying on massage tables. Variation: Draw meridians on partners using washable markers. (Figure 19-1)

- Draw areas for hara diagnosis on a student's abdomen using washable markers. (Figure 19-2).

- Demonstrate hara diagnosis and explain what you are feeling in each area. Repeat diagnosis on the back (Figure 19-3).

- Lead students through the above exercise in diagnosis.

- Show *Tappan's Handbook* CD-ROM video segment on body mechanics for Asian bodywork to accompany lecture.

- Show instructional video on Zen Shiatsu to accompany lecture.

- Demonstrate the application of shiatsu techniques on a receiver lying on a floor mat.

- Demonstrate modifications for working on a massage table.

- Lead students through practice of applying pressure on tsubos using the four principles of performing shiatsu techniques.

- Use an actual narrow neck vase and pitcher of water to illustrate principle of perpendicularity.

- Invite an experienced Zen Shiatsu practitioner to class to demonstrate the techniques and explain their application.

20

Jin Shin Do®

LECTURE OUTLINE

I. Overview and History
   A. Jin Shin Do® is a modern synthesis of traditional acupressure, breathing exercises, Taoist philosophy, and modern psychology.
   B. Jin Shin Do® is a method of releasing muscular tension and stress by applying deepening finger pressure to combinations of specific acupoints on the body.
   C. Jin Shin Do® can be translated as *the way of the compassionate spirit*.
   D. Jin Shin Do® was created by Iona Teeguarden in the 1970s.
      1. Jin Shin Do® Foundation was founded in 1982 to train, certify, and network authorized teachers.
      2. Jin Shin Do® is a registered trademark.

II. Armored Acupoints
   A. Nature of acupoints
      1. Places along energy meridians where the life force energy comes close to the surface of the body—traditional Chinese medicine.
      2. Places of high electrical conductivity or low electrical resistance compared to surrounding area—Western science
   B. Tension tends to collect at some of these points with environmental, social, emotional, or physical tension or stress.
   C. Chronic tension, called *armoring,* tends to collect at these points.
   D. Suppressed emotions or old defensive attitudes sometimes surface when tension at acupoints is released.
   E. Jin Shin Do® is *transformational* involving restoration of balance to body, mind, emotions and spirit.

III. Jin Shin Do® Technique
   A. Starts with light pressure that penetrates deeper when "invited in."
   B. Practitioner presses points for a relatively long period of time.
   C. While one hand is holding a primary tense point, the other hand holds a series of other points.
   D. Practitioners help recipients pay attention to the sensations and feelings that accompany release or armoring.
   E. Release is often accompanied by deep relaxation and occasionally by tingling, trembling, crying, or shouting.

F. Often release is followed by a new resolution and renewed ability to live joyfully.

IV. Strange Flows
   A. Strange flows, or wondrous channels, collect energy from other meridians that have excess energy.
   B. Energy does not flow continuously through strange flows, but only when energy is distributed unevenly in other meridians.
   C. Strange flows have no acupoints of their own. All their points of access are on major meridians.
   D. Strange flows are subject to armoring and blockages.
   E. A Jin Shin Do® practitioner can balance the meridians without assessing them by releasing blockages in the strange flows.
   F. There are four pairs of strange flows
      1. Yin and Yang Great Regulator Channels (GRCs)
         a. For release of shoulder and neck tension
         b. For release of nervous tension
      2. Yin and Yang Great Bridge Channels (GBCs)
         a. For release of back tension
         b. For increased energy
      3. Belt Channel (BC) and Penetrating Channel (PC)
         a. For release of abdominal and low back areas
         b. To strengthen sexual energy and organs
      4. Conception Vessel (CV) and Governing Vessel (GV)
         a. Combined are the GCC
         b. Release of GCC good for people with minor spinal or constitutional disorders, and for balancing reproductive system, especially in women *[See Figures 20-1; 20-2]*

V. Assessment of Meridians
   A. Effective Jin Shin Do® application requires assessment of which meridians and flows are imbalanced and which parts of the body are tense.
   B. Emphasis is on energetic imbalance and muscular relaxation, not on symptoms.
   C. According to Jin Shin Do® theory, the body-mind is a whole and problems in one part of the system will affect other parts as well.
   D. Assessment is focused on meridians, not physical organs.
      1. In Chinese medicine, meridians are associated with specific senses, colors, expressions, emotions, tastes, activities, as well as physical organs.
      2. Meridians are symbols and have many meanings.
      3. During a meridian's associated time or season strengths or weaknesses of the meridian are accented.
      4. Key associations of meridians *[Refer to Table 20-1]*
   E. Assessment is nonjudgmental
   F. Assessment by determining whether associated points are tense or sore
      1. Points for meridians assessment on the back *[See Figure 20-3]*
      2. Points parallel to specific vertebrae correspond to specific meridians
      3. More medial point reflects short-term problems, more lateral point indicates chronic problems
      4. Points of problem areas may be experienced as sore, numb, or spasms
   G. Once a meridian is identified, the practitioner chooses a point along the meridian to release.
      1. Primary or local point is held for about 2 minutes while other points on the meridian are pressed one after the other.
      2. Example of releasing the lung meridian *[See Figure 20-4]*

VI. Body Segments
  A. Practitioners work in body segments, or groups of muscles that are functionally related and that work together to make expressive movements or gestures.
  B. Major body segments *[See Figure 20-5]*
  C. Which body segments are tense helps the practitioner understand a recipient's emotional conflicts *[Refer to Table 20-2]*
  D. The usual procedure is to release body segments from the top down.
  E. All Jin Shin Do® sessions end with a neck release. *[See Figure 20-6]*

VII. How to Give Jin Shin Do® Sessions
  A. Main technique is finding points and pressing and holding them.
  B. The point most requiring release is called the *local point*.
  C. The local point is held while at least two other distal points are held, one after the other. Usually the points are in the same segment or on the same meridian.
  D. Pressure on a point is firm but not so deep that receiver cannot relax.
  E. As a point releases, the finger will automatically sink deeper into the tissues.
  F. Points are held for 1 or 2 minutes or until
    1. The muscle relaxes significantly.
    2. A pulse or increase in pulsation is felt.
    3. Recipient feels a decrease in sensitivity.

VIII. Benefits of Jin Shin Do®
  A. Psychological
    1. Release pent-up emotions
    2. More aware of body-mind connection
  B. Physical
    1. Release of muscular tension
    2. Reduction of stress
  C. Special populations
    1. People who cannot be moved
    2. Conditions that cannot be touched
    3. People with certain pathologies
    4. Pediatric care

SUGGESTED CLASSROOM ACTIVITIES

- Invite certified and authorized Jin Shin Do® teacher to demonstrate and explain the work to the class.

- Invite certified and authorized Jin Shin Do® teacher to teach some basic Jin Shin Do® releases to the class.

- Demonstrate a Jin Shin Do® release, explaining what you are doing and feeling during the release. Afterward, ask recipient to describe his or her experience.

- Lead students through locating a point, pressing and holding the point, and sensing a change in the point (e.g., sinking, relaxing) while holding.

- Lead students through practice of the back release (Figure 20-1), front release (Figure 20-2), lung (Figure 20-4), or neck and shoulder release (Figure 20-6).

- Lead students through meridian assessment (Figure 20-3).

21

Sports and Fitness

LECTURE OUTLINE

I. Overview
   A. Sports massage is defined as "the science and art of applying massage and related techniques to ensure the health and well-being of the athlete and to enhance athletic performance."
   B. Massage helps care for the wear and tear and minor injuries sustained in sports and fitness activities.
   C. Five major applications of sports massage
      1. Recovery
      2. Remedial
      3. Rehabilitation
      4. Maintenance
      5. Event

II. Techniques and Knowledge *[See Tappan's Handbook CD-ROM Video Segment on Sports Massage]*
   A. Sports massage is generally based in Western massage.
   B. Techniques used depend on the situation and goals of the massage
      1. Example: Compression is used in pre-event and postevent situations when athletes are clothed and increased circulation and warming of tissues is the goal. *[See Figure 21-1]*
      2. Example: Effleurage and petrissage are used more in recovery and maintenance sessions with athletes unclothed under drapes, and oil is used.
      3. Myofascial massage techniques, trigger point therapy, and lymphatic drainage are used as needed in maintenance, remedial, and rehabilitation applications.
   C. Knowledge of musculoskeletal anatomy and well-developed palpation skills help sports massage practitioners apply techniques with needed specificity.
   D. Understanding the biomechanics of sports and fitness activities helps in planning sessions and locating areas of stress.
   E. Sports massage practitioners should be well versed in the special needs of athletes and be able to adapt their massage sessions accordingly.

III. Recovery
   A. Recovery massage addresses tight, stiff, sore muscles that result from strenuous physical activity, and helps the body heal minor tissue damage.

B. Recovery is major component of maintenance sports massage.

C. Recovery massage focuses on body areas most stressed by the specific sport or physical activity.

D. Techniques used reflect goals of recovery massage
   1. Improve circulation (effleurage and petrissage)
      a. Bring nutrients to the area
      b. Flush out metabolic wastes
      c. Enhance tissue repair
   2. Promote muscular relaxation
      a. Example: joint movements [See Figure 21-2]
      b. Example: broadening techniques [See Figure 21-3]
   3. Elicit general relaxation (effleurage, light compressions)
      a. To enhance body's healing capacity
      b. Environment should be stress free with no distracting noise
      c. A hot shower, whirlpool, sauna, or steam prior to recovery massage will enhance its effects
   4. Enhance flexibility (joint movements and stretching)

IV. Remedial Massage and Rehabilitation
   A. Most common remedial and rehabilitation situations
      1. Muscle tension and loss of flexibility
      2. Muscle soreness
      3. Trigger points
      4. Edema
      5. Tendinitis
      6. Tenosynovitis
      7. Strains and sprains
      8. General stress
   B. Deep transverse friction of Cyriax friction used in rehabilitation of injuries
      1. For freeing adhesions
      2. For developing healthy scar tissue
      3. For treating tendinitis
         [See Chapter 7 section on friction techniques]
   C. Also see Myofascial Massage (Chapter 12); Neuromuscular Therapy (Chapter 13); Lymphatic Drainage Massage (Chapter 14)

V. Maintenance
   A. An all-purpose massage session received regularly that addresses the unique needs of the athlete
   B. Extra attention given to areas commonly stressed in the athlete's sport
   C. Maintenance sessions last from 60 to 90 minutes
   D. Foundation is recovery massage with remedial situations addressed.

VI. Event
   A. Event applications help the athlete prepare for and recover from specific competitive events.
   B. Includes pre-event, interevent, and postevent
      1. Pre-event
         a. Purpose is to help the athlete prepare physically and mentally for an upcoming event and may be part of a warm-up routine.
         b. Session is 15–20 minutes in duration.
         c. Upbeat in tempo
         d. Avoid causing discomfort

     e. Concentrate on major muscle groups to be used in event
     f. Adjust for psychological readiness
        1. More soothing for nervous athletes
        2. More stimulating for most athletes
     g. Athlete is usually clothed
     h. Common techniques for pre-event
        1. Compression
        2. Direct pressure on stress points
        3. Friction *[See Figure 21-4]*
        4. Lifting and broadening
        5. Percussion *[See Figure 21-5]*
        6. Jostling *[See Figure 21-6]*
        7. Joint mobilizations
        8. Stretches
2. Interevent
     a. Performed between events such as at track and swim meets
     b. Attention to recovery as well as readiness for upcoming trials
     c. Short in duration (10–15 minutes)
     d. Avoids discomfort
     e. Techniques used are combination of pre-event and postevent
        1. Example: Kneading arm *[See Figure 21-7]*
        2. Example: Shaking the arm *[See Figure 21-8]*
3. Postevent
     a. Physical and psychological recovery of athlete immediately after competition
     b. Assess injuries received during competition (for treatment, first aid, or referral)
     c. Duration of session
        1. 10–15 minutes if right after event
        2. 30–90 minutes if more than 1 hour after event
     d. Athlete should be ready for massage
        1. Cooled down
        2. Taken adequate fluids
        3. Be breathing normally
     e. Pressure lighter, pace slower that pre-event
     f. Attention to muscles used most in event
     g. Techniques for circulation, muscular relaxation, and general relaxation emphasized
        1. Compression
        2. Sliding strokes
        3. Kneading
        4. Jostling
        5. Positional release
        6. Joint movements

SUGGESTED CLASSROOM ACTIVITIES

- Show *Tappan's Handbook* CD-ROM Video Segment on Sports Massage for athletes to accompany lecture.
- Invite athletes who use massage in their training regimens to speak to the class about its benefits for them.

- Demonstrate pre-event and postevent massage on a guest athlete.
- Lead students through practice of pre-event and postevent massage.
- Make a video of massage given after an athletic event by an organized group, and show to class to accompany lecture.
- Lead students through an analysis of an athletic activity (e.g., running, bicycling, swimming, karate, bowling, golf) and its stresses and strains. As a class, or in small groups, design a 60-minute maintenance massage for an athlete in this activity.
- Invite a sports massage specialist to class to talk about their work with athletes and demonstrate their techniques.
- Arrange for "athlete's day" at a student clinic to give students the opportunity to practice maintenance sports massage.

22
Mother and Child

LECTURE OUTLINE

I. Overview
   A. Massage can relieve some of the physical and emotional stresses women experience during pregnancy.
   B. Massage is an excellent way for parents and other caregivers to provide the tactile and kinesthetic stimulation infants need for proper growth and development.

II. Pregnancy and the Benefits of Massage *[See Tappan's Handbook CD-ROM Video Segment on Pregnancy Massage]*
   A. Changes in women's bodies during pregnancy
      1. Hormonal
      2. Structural
      3. Postural
   B. Common problems
      1. Mood swings
      2. Insomnia
      3. Swelling of hands, legs, and feet
      4. Strain on lower back
      5. Instability and pain in joints from softening of connective tissue, including cartilage and ligaments, during pregnancy
   C. Typical pregnancy posture *[See Figure 22-1]*
      1. Head forward
      2. Chest back
      3. Belly out
      4. Hips tilted forward
      5. Locked knees
      6. Feet turned out
   D. Intent of pregnancy massage
      1. Relaxation
      2. Release emotional stress
      3. Relieve strain in lower back, neck, legs, and feet
      4. Reduce edema in extremities
      5. Research shows potential for reducing complications of pregnancy including lower prematurity rates.

III. Contraindications and Cautions for Pregnancy Massage
  A. Best to get permission from woman's health care provider before massage
  B. Abdominal massage is contraindicated during pregnancy, with possible exception of nerve strokes, passive touch, and some forms of energy work.
  C. General contraindications
    1. Morning sickness
    2. Nausea or vomiting
    3. Vaginal bleeding or discharge
    4. Fever
    5. Decrease in fetal movement over past 24 hours
    6. Diarrhea
    7. Pain in the abdomen or anywhere else in the body
    8. Excessive swelling in the arms or legs
    9. Immediately after eating (wait two hours)
    10. Over a bruise or skin irritation (local contraindication)
  D. Chinese medicine contraindications
    1. Avoid strong pressure over the Gall Bladder Channel at the tops of the shoulders, and acupoints L14 and Sp6.
    2. If worry about miscarriage, avoid pressure on Yin channels in the inside of the lower legs.
IV. Pregnancy Massage Set-Up
  A. Environment
    1. Keep room 5–10 degrees cooler than usual for massage
    2. Provide good air flow and fresh air
    3. Bathroom readily available
    4. Relaxing atmosphere
    5. Glass of water in reach for recipient
    6. Tissues handy
  B. Massage table and positioning
    1. Set table height lower than usual for good body mechanics
    2. Have several bolsters and pillows available to prop up client
    3. Provide stable stepping stool for recipient to get onto the table
    4. Assist recipient onto the table if necessary
  C. Positioning options
    1. In first few months, women may be comfortable prone or supine.
    2. Once belly gets larger other options for positioning may be better.
        a. Later in pregnancy lying supine is not desirable.
          1. Fetus puts pressure on descending aorta impeding blood flow to placenta and causing shortness of breath
          2. Pressure on vena cave resulting in light-headedness, nausea or backache
        b. Lying prone is usually uncomfortable.
    3. Reclining, or half-sitting, may be good alternative.
    4. Side-lying is most common positioning alternative
  D. Positioning procedure
    1. General rule of thumb: Whatever the position is, fill in spaces between the body and the table with bolsters, pillows, or rolled-up towels.
    2. In supine or reclining positions, use bolster under knees.
    3. In prone position, bolster under shoulders, ankles, and around belly.
    4. In side-lying position, pillows are placed in several places. *[See Figure 22-2]*
        a. Under and around the belly

   b. Under the top arm

   c. Under the top leg or between the legs

   d. Under the head

  5. Draping for side-lying position *[See Figure 22-3]*

V. Pregnancy Massage Session

 A. General qualities: gentle and relaxing

 B. Special attention to neck, chest, lower back, hips, legs, and feet

 C. Neck and back can be accessed in side-lying position.

  1. Example: Massage of upper back *[See Figure 22-4]*

  2. Example: Massage of neck *[See Figure 22-5]*

 D. Suggestions for massage

  1. Address tension in upper back and neck.

  2. Attention to muscles of respiration can enhance breathing.

  3. Relieve tension in the lower back with firm effleurage in side-lying position.

  4. Distal to proximal effleurage on lower extremities can move fluids out.

  5. Avoid deep pressure on inner thighs.

  6. Massage the feet.

 E. Labor, delivery, recovery

  1. Midwives, childbirth assistants, and others in the delivery room may use massage during labor and delivery to assist the process.

   a. As simple as stroking the mother's hand

   b. Massage has been shown to reduce anxiety and labor pain.

   c. Massage may decrease the length of labor and need for medication.

   d. Acupressure points to relieve labor pain include Shoulder Well (GB21) on the trapezius; Sacral Points (GB 27–34); Hoku (L14) on the thumb web; Bigger Stream (K3) near Achilles Tendon; Reaching Inside (B67) on the little toe.

  2. Recovery after labor

   a. Traditional Western massage can help relax stressed and sore muscles and relax nerves.

   b. Acupressure points for postpartum recovery include Sea of Energy (CV6) just below the navel; Inner Gate (P6) inside of the forearm above the wrist; Sea of Vitality (B23 and B47) back at waist level; Womb and Vitals (B48) lateral to sacrum; Three Mile Point (St36) on lower leg; Bigger rushing (Lv3) on top of the foot.

  3. After C-section and after enough healing time has taken place, massage around scar tissue can help address adhesions and healthy scar formation.

 F. Women with infants and toddlers

  1. Massage affords an opportunity to take time out and relax.

  2. Can address the stress on the upper back and arms from picking up, holding, and nursing growing babies.

  3. Breast massage may be useful for relieving the discomforts of nursing.

VI. Benefits of Infant Massage

 A. A significant amount of research shows that massage is beneficial for infants

  1. Contributes to healthy development of normal infants

  2. Facilitates recovery and development of high risk infants (e.g., preterm, cocaine exposed, HIV exposed)

 B. General benefits of infant massage

  1. Releasing tension and learning to relax

  2. Bonding with parents and caregivers

  3. Aiding digestion and elimination

4. Improving sleep
5. Easing growing pains
6. Calming colicky babies
C. Mothers and fathers
   1. Promotes milk production in the mother by stimulating secretion of prolactin
   2. Provides an opportunity for fathers to touch and interact with their infants in a way that builds confidence in handling the child

VII. Infant Massage Session *[See Tappan's Handbook CD-ROM Video Segment on Infant Massage]*
   A. Simple, gentle, yet firm application of stroking, pressing, squeezing, and movement of the arms and legs.
   B. Maintain eye contact throughout the massage when infant is supine.
   C. Talk or sing to child during the massage.
   D. Time for social interaction that helps infants emotional and social development.
   E. Techniques can be practiced by caregivers on dolls before delivery.
   F. Sample techniques
      1. Gentle circles on the head *[See Figure 22-6]*
      2. Effleurage diagonally on chest *[See Figure 22-7]*
      3. Thumb strokes to hands *[See Figure 22-8]*
      4. Thumb strokes to feet *[See Figure 22-9]*
      5. Effleurage over abdomen *[See Figure 22-10]*
      6. Long stroke over backs of legs *[See Figure 22-11]*
      7. Arm movement across chest *[See Figure 22-12]*
      8. Knees to abdomen *[See Figure 22-13]*
      9. Squeeze and twist on legs *[See Figure 22-14]*

SUGGESTED CLASSROOM ACTIVITIES

- Show *Tappan's Handbook* CD-ROM Video Segment on Pregnancy Massage to accompany lecture.

- Show instructional video on pregnancy massage to accompany lecture.

- Invite a pregnant woman to class to be model for pregnancy massage demonstration. Ask her to talk about the problems she is experiencing related to the pregnancy before the demonstration.

- Students practice set-up for pregnancy massage and working with recipient in side-lying position.

- Invite a midwife or childbirth assistant to class to discuss the use of massage during labor and delivery.

- Borrow a "pregnant suit" or similar device so that students can experience carrying the extra weight of carrying a child and feel how it affects their posture. Variation: Have students assume the typical posture of a pregnant woman without props to see how it stresses the body.

- Arrange a "pregnant women's day" at student clinic so that students can practice pregnancy massage. Screen participants beforehand for contraindications and appropriateness for student massage.

- Lead students through a practice of infant massage on dolls.

- Invite a caregiver and his or her infant to class and teach infant massage. The class watches the demonstration.

- Show *Tappan's Handbook* CD-ROM Video segment on Infant Massage to accompany lecture.

23

Healthy Aging

LECTURE OUTLINE

I. Overview
   A. Regular massage can be an important component of life-long wellness.
   B. Massage addresses conditions commonly associated with aging and enhances the quality of life.
   C. Massage works best as a measure of prevention.

II. Effects of Aging and Benefits of Massage
   A. Physical effects of aging are noticeable starting by age 30 for most.
      1. Decrease in general mobility and strength
      2. Slower nerve conduction
      3. Less efficient circulation
      4. Less tissue elasticity
      5. Thinner and dryer skin
      6. Loss of bone mass
      7. Decreased function of the senses (sight, hearing, smell, taste)
      8. Less efficient immune system
      9. Experienced as general aches and pains, slower movement, and less stamina
   B. Many of the above "biomarkers" can be slower with healthy lifestyle.
   C. Massage addresses many effects of aging directly.
      1. Promotes well-nourished skin
         a. Increases superficial circulation
         b. Moisturizes skin with oils and lotions
      2. Improves general blood circulation
      3. Improves lymphatic and immune system function
      4. Reduces the physical and mental effects of chronic stress
      5. Relieves stiff sore muscles
      6. Helps maintain flexibility
   D. Special benefits for elders (over 65 years)
      1. Helps maintain independence and with activities of daily living (ADL)
      2. Improves digestion and elimination *[See Figure 23-1]*
      3. Helps ease pain of loss of work, home, family, friends, etc.

4. Provides an avenue of social interaction
    a. Reduces feelings of social isolation
    b. Touch provides essential connection to others
5. Other benefits
    a. Relieves insomnia
    b. Helps improve appetite
    c. Improves mobility
    d. Improves circulation, especially important for less active people
    e. Improves immune system function
    f. Improves skin condition
    g. Helps prevent pressure sores
    h. Relieves physical discomfort and pain
    i. Relieves chronic pain and stress
    j. Relieves feeling alone and useless
6. Research on massage and the elderly *[See Figure 23-2]*
    a. Massage beneficial for reducing anxiety of hospitalized elders
    b. Back massage to institutionalized elders provides relaxation, improved communication, and reduction in dehumanizing effects of institutionalized care
    c. Promising research on massage as beneficial for agitated elderly and those with Alzheimer's disease and dementia.
       1. Short sessions of 10 minutes
       2. Light pressure, even rhythm, slow strokes

III. Working with the Elderly
   A. General characteristics
      1. Elders are more different from each other than any other age group.
      2. Elders have accumulated a lifetime of good and poor health habits, diseases and injuries, and life experiences.
      3. Elders are more likely to have chronic health problems.
      4. Elders are more likely to be on medication.
   B. Physiological age categories (versus chronological age)
      1. *Robust elders* have few outward signs of impaired health.
         a. Look younger than their age
         b. Mentally sharp and physically active
         c. For massage, treat like typical middle-aged adult
         d. Identify hidden massage cautions from health history
      2. *Age appropriate elders* show some of the typical signs of aging.
         a. Identify massage cautions and medications from health history.
         b. Use bolstering to ensure maximum comfort and relieve stress on joints.
         c. Limit prone position to 15–20 minutes.
         d. Help recipient sit up after massage if necessary, or at least stay until he or she is sitting up.
         e. Leave the room only when you are sure that recipient is not light-headed and can get off of the table safely.
      3. *Frail elders* have significant loss of function, are weak, and have limited mobility.
         a. Check with physician before massaging the very frail.
         b. Help frail elders getting on and off the massage table.
         c. Massage in bed or chair if unable to get onto table safely.
         d. Limit sessions to 15–20 minutes until you know that the elder can benefit from longer sessions.

  e. Watch carefully in prone position to be sure that the elder can lie there comfortably.

  f. Be extra gentle in lifting frail elders; avoid pulling on their arms to help them up.

  g. Cradle their bodies to help them change position.

 C. Seated massage for the elderly

  1. Use good body mechanics for your own safety

  2. Examples of seated massage techniques:

   a. Massage of head *[See Figure 23-3]*

   b. Massage of hands *[See Figure 23-4*

   c. Massage of feet *[See Figure 23-5]*

IV. Guidelines for Massage for Healthy Aging *[See Tappan's Handbook CD-ROM Video Segment on Massage for the Elderly]*

 A. *Do* include the following:

  1. Techniques to improve circulation in extremities

  2. Techniques to keep muscles and connective tissues pliable and elastic

  3. Joint movements for improved flexibility and mobility

  4. Joint movements of the hands, arms, and shoulders to help maintain ability to perform activities of daily living

  5. Passive range of motion and stretches for neck

  6. Techniques to lengthen the front of the body for erect posture

  7. Abdominal massage for digestion and elimination

 B. Cautions *[See Tappan's Handbook Chapter 5 Endangerment Sites, Contraindications, Cautions]*

  1. Take note of medications and observe appropriate precautions.

  2. Use gentle to moderate pressure and sufficient lubricant for thin, delicate skin.

  3. Watch for varicose veins and avoid pressure over them.

  4. Avoid deep work in lateral neck, or movements that put neck in hyperextension or increase the cervical curve.

  5. Identify those with joint replacements and limit joint movements as appropriate.

  6. Check with physician before performing massage on someone with cancer.

  7. Avoid areas of inflammation, especially around joints.

  8. Look out for suspicious skin lesions that might be cancer. Report to recipient or caregiver, and avoid massage over the site.

SUGGESTED CLASSROOM ACTIVITIES

- Show *Tappan's Handbook* CD-ROM Video Segment on Massage for the Elderly to accompany lecture.

- Show instructional video on massage for the aging and elderly to accompany lecture. Variation: Show instructional video on geriatrics or elders in nursing homes for background information.

- Invite an elderly person to class for demonstration of adaptations of massage to meet his or her needs. Variation: Invite older people from each of the physiological age categories to class to illustrate the differences in approach to massage for each group.

- Arrange a "healthy aging day" at student clinic for students to practice giving massage to the elderly.

- Student presentations of case studies of elders with whom they have been practicing massage and applying information from the chapter

24

Terminally Ill and Dying

LECTURE OUTLINE

I. Overview
   A. Simple massage techniques can be used by health practitioners and taught to nonprofessional caregivers to aid the serious ill or those approaching the end of their lives.
   B. Massage is a valuable complementary therapy in hospitals, hospice, and home care.

II. The Caring Touch of Massage
   A. From the wellness perspective, even those with terminal illness or nearing death continue to strive for optimal well-being in their life circumstances.
      1. Massage can help improve physical functioning and ease pain, anxiety, and discomfort.
      2. Massage provides multiple psychosocial, mental, emotional, and physical benefits.
      3. Nurturing touch provides food for the soul as well as the body and mind.
   B. Specific benefits of massage for the terminally ill and those who have been inactive or bedridden for a long period of time:
      1. Improved circulation, reduced muscular tension, general relaxation
      2. Stimulates receptors in skin
      3. Alleviates problems with insomnia, digestion, constipation, breathing difficulties, and skin degeneration
      4. Alleviates feelings of isolation, fear, and depression
      5. Relieves touch deprivation
      6. Reduces anxiety, facilitates release of pent-up feelings, frustrations, sadness, and emotional energy
      7. Provides a sense of connection
      8. Helps reduce pain

III. Hospice and Palliative Care
   A. Hospice and palliative care facilities
      1. Freestanding facilities
      2. In hospitals
      3. Nursing homes
      4. Long-term care facilities
   B. Team-oriented approach to patient care
      1. Medical care

2. Pain management
3. Emotional and spiritual support
C. Hospice service goal is to provide high-quality palliative care
    1. Nursing care
    2. Personal care
    3. Social services
    4. Physician visits
    5. Counseling
    6. Domestic services
D. The value of massage as palliative care has been studies and validated in integrative medical settings

IV. Massage for the Dying [See Tappan's Handbook CD-ROM Video Segment on Massage for the Terminally Ill and Dying]
A. Massage provides an avenue of nonverbal communicaton.
    1. Quality of touch should be gentle
    2. Techniques should be simple (e.g., stroking and holding)
B. Example: TLP (Tender Loving Physiotherapy) Program in New Zealand
    1. Short-term rehabilitation and clearing the chest
    2. Easing transition from life to death
    3. Provides soothing touch as a form of comfort and communication
C. Example: Therapeutic Touch used with the dying
    1. Placing hands over or near the heart
    2. Consciously sending thoughts of peace, love, wholeness
    3. Helps decrease predeath anxiety
    4. Elders report feelings of warmth, peace, and calm
D. Benefits for caregivers who perform massage
    1. Offers caregivers something active to do
    2. Provides means of nonverbal connection and communication

V. Massage Skills and Other Abilities
A. Medical profile of recipient is essential
    1. Identify contraindications and areas of caution
    2. Understand symptoms expected as disease or condition progresses
B. Specific techniques are less important than other essential abilities
    1. Seeing the individual
    2. Reaching out with caring and open heart
    3. Intuition and sensitivity
    4. Being touch oriented
    5. Ability to adapt
    6. Openhearted
    7. Ability to focus energy
    8. Willing to face death
C. Helpful skills related to massage
    1. Perform sensitive massage
    2. Active holding
    3. Listening and feedback
    4. Visualization and guided fantasy
    5. Guided meditation
    6. Shared breathing
    7. Communicating with the dying

D. General guidelines for massage with terminally ill
   1. Sessions are softer, gentler, shorter.
   2. 10–20 minutes of contact
   3. Techniques vary from hand holding to full-body massage.
   4. Recipient on massage table, or on a chair or wheel chair, or lying in bed.
   5. Recipient may be in a hospital bed with tubes or hooked to intravenous (IV) tubes.
   6. Massage practitioners should be versatile and adaptable.
   7. Be caring, supportive, and accepting.
   8. Hand and arm massage is a useful approach.
      a. Hands are easily accessible, relatively safe area for massage
      b. Hands benefit from application of lotion
      c. Hands are a familiar place of contact with other people
      d. Having hands touched is comforting
      e. Hand massage allows eye contact while talking

VI. Self-Care
   A. Physical self-care
      1. Techniques used are simple and light and so usually easy on the hands.
      2. Use good body mechanics especially when recipients are in chairs or beds.
      3. Use appropriate precautions to protect yourself from communicable disease (e.g., good hygiene and latex or similar gloves).
   B. Emotional self-care
      1. Confront your own issues and fears about illness and death to a point of acceptance.
      2. Work through feelings with a friend, co-worker or supervisor.
      3. When a client dies, be sensitive to your own process of grieving.
      4. Use ongoing professional supervision or peer counseling.

SUGGESTED CLASSROOM ACTIVITIES

- Show *Tappan's Handbook* CD-ROM Video Segment on Massage for the Terminally Ill and Dying to accompany lecture.

- Show instructional video on caring for the terminally ill or on hospices to accompany lecture.

- Students practice hand and arm massage with recipient sitting in a chair. Variation: With recipients in wheel chairs or hospital beds.

- Arrange a field trip to a nursing home to provide massage for residents.

- Invite a local hospice director or other worker to class to talk about the hospice and its approach to palliative care.

25

Seated Massage in the Workplace

LECTURE OUTLINE

I. Overview
  A. Massage is increasingly popular in workplace wellness programs.
  B. Seated massage in particular is popular with businesses exploring ways to reduce stress in the workplace, minimize job-related injuries, and increase productivity.

II. History of Workplace Massage
  A. In late nineteenth and early twentieth centuries, massage was often available at the workplace.
    1. Industrial recreation programs
    2. On-site medical services including physiotherapy
    3. Massage on-site for executives
    4. Largely disappeared by mid-twentieth century
  B. In 1980s workplace wellness revived as a concept.
    1. Typical wellness programs included exercise, weight loss, smoking cessation, and stress reduction.
    2. Programs found to reduce workers' compensation claims and absenteeism.
  C. Invention of special massage chair helped bring massage back to the workplace.
    1. First modern massage chair was designed by David Palmer of San Francisco in mid-1980s.
    2. The original idea of the massage chair was to make receiving massage more accessible to the general public.
      a. Can be used in public places
      b. Recipients get massage sitting up with clothes on
      c. Originally used for amma (traditional Japanese massage) but can be adapted for any massage that can be done over clothing
    3. One of first large corporations to provide on-site massage was Apple Computer Corporation in 1985.

III. Benefits of Massage in the Workplace
  A. Reduces incidence of repetitive strain injuries (RSIs)
    1. Computer keyboard work
    2. Sorting, filing, assembly-line tasks

B. Relieves effects of poor posture and workspace ergonomics
  1. Sitting for long periods of time at workstations
  2. Sitting at computers for long periods of time
C. Lowers stress level of employees
  1. Helps prevent burnout
  2. Helps reduce stress-related diseases
  3. Addresses tension headache and stiff sore muscles
D. Improves immune function for more resistance to illness
E. Increases mental clarity and alertness
  1. Improves ability to focus
  2. Antidote for workday slumps
F. Increases worker productivity with employees revitalized and ready to return to work

IV. Seated Massage for Office Workers *[See Tappan's Handbook CD-ROM Video Segment on Seated Massage for the Workplace]*
  A. Seated massage can be adapted for a variety of spaces.
    1. At a workstation
    2. In an empty office or cubicle
    3. Corner of conference room or workroom
  B. Duration is 15–20 minutes.
  C. Equipment
    1. Table-top massage set-up *[See Figure 25-1]*
    2. Regular chairs
    3. Special massage chairs
  D. Recipient is clothed.
    1. Remove large jewelry
    2. Remove jacket and tie
    3. Ask permission to work on face or scalp.
  E. Focus of seated massage is on upper body (i.e., neck and shoulders, head and scalp, upper back, forearms, hands).
  F. Techniques that can be performed over clothing are used:
    1. Compression, direct pressure, kneading, friction, tapotement, light stroking, joint movements
    2. Passive touch, holding, and energy techniques
    3. Asian bodywork such as amma and shiatsu
  G. Examples of techniques
    1. Kneading the shoulders *[See Figure 25–2]*
    2. Direct pressure to paraspinal muscles *[See Figure 25–3]*
    3. Hand, wrist, and forearm massage *[See Figure 25–4]*
    4. Neck massage *[See Figure 25–5]*
    5. Circular friction to the head and scalp *[See Figure 25–6]*
    6. Light tapotement to the head *[See Figure 25–7]*

V. Popularity of Workplace Massage
  A. Immediate positive effects since workers feel better right away.
  B. Alleviates some of the aches and pains of sitting long hours at a workstation.
  C. Massage requires no practice or effort on the part of the recipient.
  D. Massage complements other health practices such as exercise, stress reduction, and weight reduction programs.
  E. Workplace massage helps increase good feeling about and loyalty to the employer.
  F. Boosts productivity and may be taken advantage of by most workers.

SUGGESTED CLASSROOM ACTIVITIES

- Show *Tappan's Handbook* CD-ROM Video Segment on Seated Massage for the Workplace to accompany lecture.
- Demonstrate 15-minute seated massage routine for the workplace.
- Lead students through a practice of a seated massage routine for the workplace.
- Students observe a 15-minute seated massage session and evaluate the body mechanics of the practitioner. Discuss the similarities to and differences from table massage.
- Arrange for field trip to a business to provide complimentary seated massage to employees.
- Invite to class a massage practitioner whose main practice is workplace massage. Ask him or her to describe his or her practice, the workplace environment, and the type of massage he or she offers. Have him or her demonstrate the massage for the class.

Test Bank

CHAPTER 1 HEALING MASSAGE—A WELLNESS PERSPECTIVE

1. The chief aim of natural healing methods is to enhance the
   a. medical treatment.
   b. curing of patients.
   c. innate healing force.
   d. prescribed medication.

2. Which characteristics are associated with the idea of *healing*?
   a. outside force, passive recipient
   b. outside force, active recipient
   c. inside force, passive recipient
   d. inside force, active recipient

3. The term *massage and bodywork* describes
   a. categories of Western massage.
   b. a wide variety of manual therapies.
   c. Asian bodywork therapy.
   d. holistic approach to healing.

4. The actions and intentions of the practitioner constitute the
   a. massage technique.
   b. Ayurvedic massage tradition.
   c. natural healing philosophy.
   d. wellness perspective.

5. Lomi-lomi of Hawaii is an example of the _____ massage tradition.
   a. native and folk
   b. Ayurvedic
   c. Asian bodywork
   d. Western massage and bodywork

6. The Ayurvedic massage tradition originated in
   a. China.
   b. the United States.
   c. Sweden.
   d. India.

7. The following is *not* one of the seven major Western massage technique categories.
   a. effleurage
   b. polarity
   c. friction
   d. joint movements

8. Percussion techniques, like rapping and cupping, fall into the following major Western massage technique category.
   a. effleurage
   b. petrissage
   c. tapotement
   d. friction

9. Passive touch, holding, and laying the hands on the body are examples of the following major Western massage technique category.
   a. petrissage
   b. tapotement
   c. friction
   d. touch without movement

10. One of the following is *not* considered a form of contemporary massage and bodywork.
    a. lymphatic drainage massage
    b. Ayurvedic massage
    c. neuromuscular massage
    d. polarity therapy

11. Practitioners who incorporate elements of different traditions or systems of massage and bodywork are called
    a. eclectic.
    b. holistic.
    c. integrative.
    d. alternative.

12. The following term is used when a prescribed healing method is considered secondary to the treatments of mainstream medicine.
    a. alternative
    b. complementary
    c. integrative
    d. eclectic

13. The International Spa Association (ISPA) identifies a category for spas that integrate spa services with conventional and complementary therapies. These are called
    a. destination spas.
    b. day spas.
    c. specialty spas.
    d. medical spas.

14. A wellness perspective goes beyond the old idea of health as the absence of disease to the goal of achieving
    a. injury and disease prevention.
    b. a vibrant, meaningful life.
    c. recovery from disease or injury.
    d. a pain- and disease-free existence.

15. On Travis's Illness/Wellness Continuum, the halfway marker on the continuum is
    a. signs and symptoms.
    b. awareness point.
    c. neutral point.
    d. high-level wellness.

16–21. Match the following activities with the most appropriate Component of Wellness and a Healthy Lifestyle:

_____ 16. seeking counsel when needed
_____ 17. having a network of family and friends
_____ 18. knowing your purpose in life
_____ 19. getting adequate sleep
_____ 20. school and job satisfaction
_____ 21. learning from life experiences

    a. physical well-being
    b. emotional well-being
    c. intellectual well-being
    d. social well-being
    e. spiritual well-being
    f. vocational well-being

22. The Wellness Massage Pyramid is a useful tool for describing
    a. the reasons people seek massage.
    b. physical well-being.
    c. the treatment model.
    d. natural healing philosophy.

23. The three levels at the base of the Wellness Massage Pyramid that represent deficiency needs are
    a. health maintenance, personal growth, and enjoyment of life.
    b. prevention, neutral zone, and health maintenance.
    c. recovery, prevention, and personal growth.
    d. treatment, recovery, and prevention.

24. Seeking massage to relieve self-diagnosed muscular stress from repetitive motion would be considered to be at this level of the Wellness Massage Pyramid.
    a. treatment
    b. prevention
    c. neural zone
    d. personal growth

25. The following terms are wellness terminology.
    a. patient, rehabilitation, and protocol
    b. client, assessment, and session strategy
    c. case, diagnosis, and intervention
    d. case history, treatment plan, and medical setting

Short Answer and Essay Questions

26. Explain the difference between the concepts of *healing* and *curing*. Why is the concept of *healing* a better fit for the natural healing arts and philosophy?

27. Name and describe the four major massage and bodywork traditions. Give examples of each.

28. Name and describe the seven basic Western massage technique categories. Give an example of a specific massage technique for each category.

29. Discuss the relationship between conventional Western medicine and therapies that are called *alternative* and *complementary*. Explain the concept of *integrative health care* and how it differs from that of *CAM* therapies. Use examples from massage therapy in your discussion.

30. Draw the Wellness Pyramid, labeling the levels from bottom to top. Use the Wellness Pyramid to explain the many different reasons people seek massage. Be specific in your examples.

CHAPTER 2 A HISTORY OF MASSAGE

1. Maori of New Zealand had a tradition of treating club feet in infants with continuous massage of the feet performed by
   a. assigned tribal healers.
   b. Western doctors.
   c. older women in the family.
   d. young warriors.

2. A clay tablet from Sumer (2100 B.C.E.) describes "rubbing" and "friction" as a remedy to be used with
   a. an herbal mixture.
   b. exercise.
   c. tuina.
   d. bone setting.

3. *The Yellow Emperor's Classic of Internal Medicine* (c. 500 B.C.E.) describes the essential concepts of traditional
   a. Western medicine.
   b. Greek medicine.
   c. Japanese medicine.
   d. Chinese medicine.

4. This man developed shiatsu in Japan in the 1940s.
   a. Torujiro Namikoshi
   b. Pehr Ling
   c. Yellow Emperor
   d. Sobardora

5. Ayur-veda, the name of traditional medicine of India, means
   a. balanced energy.
   b. cleansing charkas.
   c. knowledge of long life.
   d. knowledge of doshas.

6. This famous Greek physician wrote about *frictions* for the treatment of sprains and dislocations.
   a. Aristotle
   b. Hippocrates
   c. Alexander the Great
   d. Galen

7. Massage given at the gymnasia of ancient Athens and Sparta was characterized by the liberal use of
   a. oil.
   b. towels.
   c. joint cracking.
   d. sand.

8. The Roman writer Seneca (4 B.C.E.–65 C.E.) commented on this feature of the massage given at the Roman baths.
   a. slippery oil
   b. dry rubbing
   c. noisy percussion
   d. relaxing silence

9. In the 1500s, this founder of modern surgery wrote about the use of frictions for joint stiffness and wound healing.
   a. Avicenna
   b. Ambrose Pare
   c. Seneca
   d. Celsus

10. Pehr H. Ling (1776–1839) developed a system of active and passive movements for treating a variety of ailments that he called
    a. Swedish massage.
    b. Swedish movements.
    c. medical gymnastics.
    d. medical massage.

11. In the United States, Ling's system was called
    a. Swedish movement cure.
    b. physical culture.
    c. wellness movement.
    d. holistic massage.

12. The physician from Amsterdam who popularized the classic massage technique categories using French terminology (e.g., effleurage) was
    a. Ambrose Pare.
    b. C. M. Sampson.
    c. Johann Mezger.
    d. H. Joseph Fay.

13. This early pioneer of physiotherapy, from the Training School of St. Thomas Hospital in London, stressed care and gentleness in giving massage and wrote an influential text about his approach to massage in 1917.
    a. Albert Hoffa
    b. James B. Mennell
    c. Douglas Graham
    d. Kurre Ostrom

14. This pioneer of physical therapy in the United States was an instructor of the war emergency course for reconstruction aides in World War I and became Director of Physiotherapy at Harvard Medical School in 1921.
    a. Albert Hoffa
    b. James B. Mennell
    c. C. W. Post
    d. Mary McMillan

15. Swedish massage is a genre of massage that historically has included adjunct therapies such as
    a. herbal remedies.
    b. Swedish movements and hydrotherapy.
    c. amma and shiatsu.
    d. biologic living.

16. The Battle Creek Sanitarium in Michigan was a well-known natural healing resort in the late nineteenth century. Its famous director, who also invented breakfast cereal, was
    a. C. W. Post.
    b. Mary McMillan.
    c. J. Harvey Kellogg.
    d. Bernarr MacFadden.

17. This promoter popularized natural healing, including massage, as *physical culture* through magazines, radio shows, and health resorts (early 1900s).
    a. C. W. Post
    b. J. Harvey Kellogg
    c. Bernarr MacFadden
    d. Harry Andrews

18. The mainstay of massage for athletes in the late nineteenth century was
    a. the rubdown.
    b. physcultapathy.
    c. Swedish massage.
    d. Mennell's massage.

19. A sensual form of Western massage developed in California, and popularized in the 1970s as part of the human potential movement, was called
    a. Swedish massage.
    b. Esalen massage.
    c. Ayurvedic massage.
    d. Tuina.

20. What year saw several advances for massage therapy, including the incorporation of the AMTA Foundation, the founding of the Touch Research Institute, and the first National Certification Examination for Therapeutic Massage and Bodywork?
    a. 1963
    b. 1975
    c. 1984
    d. 1992

Short Answer and Essay Questions

21. Describe the uses of massage in the ancient civilizations of China, India, Greece, and Rome. Give approximate dates (e.g., circa 500 B.C.E.) and one or two examples of how massage was used in each society.

22. Trace the early development of Western massage and the contributions of Pehr H. Ling and Johann Mezger. Include approximate dates and terminology used at the time.

23. Discuss the development of massage in the early twentieth century as used in physical therapy. Include important people and their contributions and approximate dates.

24. Discuss the natural healing movement of the late nineteenth and early twentieth centuries. Trace its origin, philosophy, people, institutions, and the types and uses of massage within that context.

25. Describe the revival of interest in massage in the 1970s. Include the contributions of the counterculture, human potential movement, the Esalen Institute, and the wellness movement.

26. Discuss the professionalization of massage in the 1990s. Include the major milestones.

CHAPTER 3 EFFECTS AND BENEFITS OF MASSAGE

1. Practitioners who can apply techniques to produce specific effects will be more successful in achieving
   a. good body mechanics.
   b. session or treatment goals.
   c. hygienic conditions.
   d. relaxing environment.

2. Massage is contraindicated in the immediate location of an injury during the _____ phase of tissue healing.
   a. inflammatory
   b. regeneration
   c. remodeling
   d. lymphatic

3. Cyriax or transverse friction is applied in the remodeling phase of tissue healing to enhance
   a. inflammation.
   b. local circulation.
   c. healthy scar formation.
   d. removal of excess fluid.

4. Connective tissue becomes more fluid and pliable when it is mobile and firmer when less mobile. This characteristic is called
   a. fibrosis.
   b. regeneration.
   c. approximation.
   d. thixotropy.

5. Body awareness and pain reduction are the result of stimulation of these structures in the skin.
   a. sebaceous glands
   b. hair follicles
   c. sensory receptors
   d. connective tissue

6. Petrissage massage techniques mimic _____, helping to minimize the effects of under- or overactivity.
   a. muscle contraction
   b. relaxation response
   c. respiration
   d. flexibility

7. Which of the following is *not* a primary mechanism for muscle relaxation during massage?
   a. relaxation response
   b. conscious letting go of tension
   c. decrease in T-cells
   d. increased sensory stimulation

8. Which of the following is *not* a primary goal during applications of massage to increase flexibility at a joint?
   a. relax hypertonic muscles
   b. increase activity of sebaceous glands
   c. deactivate trigger points
   d. increase connective tissue pliablity

9. Warm and red skin after superficial friction is a sign of
    a. hyperemia.
    b. thixotropy.
    c. blood clots.
    d. metabolic waste.

10. Deep stroking in the limbs should always be performed
    a. proximal to distal.
    b. distal to proximal.
    c. horizontal.
    d. vertical.

11. A condition in which normal blood flow in veins is slowed or halted is called
    a. hyperemia.
    b. vessel dilation.
    c. hypertension.
    d. venostasis.

12. Massage has been shown to _____ the number of red blood cells in circulation.
    a. increase
    b. decrease
    c. stabilize
    d. deactivate

13. Movement of lymph fluid through lymphatic vessels is largely dependent on
    a. heart action.
    b. muscle contractions.
    c. relaxation.
    d. blood pressure.

14. Which of the following effects of massage is an indication of improved immune function?
    a. reduced blood pressure
    b. muscle relaxation
    c. decreased blood cortisol levels
    d. enhanced deep breathing

15. Which of the following statements about a client's penis erection during massage is true?
    a. An erection is always a sign of sexual arousal.
    b. An erection may be the result of increased blood flow from massage.
    c. If an erection occurs, the session should be ended immediately.
    d. An erection is natural and should always be ignored.

16. Desired traits such as calmness, gentleness, and nonaggressiveness have been associated with _____ in early life.
    a. stimulating kinesthetic experiences
    b. good digestive function
    c. adequate lymphatic flow
    d. adequate pleasurable tactile experiences

17. Which of the following would *not* be appropriate during relaxation massage?
    a. techniques that cause discomfort
    b. flowing effleurage techniques
    c. warm room temperature
    d. petrissage techniques

18. Which of the following types of massage works best for increased mental clarity?
    a. one-hour relaxation massage
    b. lymphatic drainage massage
    c. 20-minute chair massage
    d. deep transverse friction massage

19. Release of endorphins associated with massage would have which of the following effects?
    a. muscle relaxation
    b. improved lymph flow
    c. break fascial adhesions
    d. increased feeling of well-being

20. Physical forces such as compression, stretching, shearing, and broadening of tissues are behind the _____ effects of massage.
    a. mechanical
    b. physiological
    c. reflex
    d. energetic

21. The new science of _____ has grown from the study of body-mind effects on health and disease.
    a. mechano-therapeutic-ology
    b. psycho-neuro-immunology
    c. psycho-reflex-ornothology
    d. reflex-neuro-immunology

22. Function changes mediated by the nervous system are considered
    a. mechanical effects.
    b. reflex effects.
    c. energetic effects.
    d. mind-body effects.

23. The term used to describe the body-mind working as a single unit is
    a. holistic.
    b. body-centered.
    c. limbic.
    d. biomedical.

24. A group of structures within the brain associated with emotions and feelings is called the _____ system.
    a. neurological
    b. parasympathetic
    c. embryonic
    d. limbic

25. Muscular tension caused by unexpressed emotions is called
    a. body-centered.
    b. mechanical.
    c. character armor.
    d. hypertonic.

Short Answer and Essay Questions

26. Explain the three phases of the process of tissue repair. Discuss the uses of massage to facilitate the process, including the contraindications and goals, and specific techniques appropriate for each phase.

27. Explain four different ways that massage is used to elicit muscle relaxation. Include descriptions of specific massage techniques.

28. Discuss the contributions of massage to the healthy functioning of *one* of the following body systems: cardiovascular, lymphatic, or integumentary.

29. Explain the use massage for wellness related to *one* of the following organism-level phenomena: growth and development, pain, or stress. Describe specific massage techniques where applicable.

30. Explain the benefits of massage for psychological well-being. Include at least three specific effects and massage forms or techniques where applicable.

31. Name and describe five mechanisms used to explain how the effects of massage are produced. Give an example of each mechanism.

32. Discuss *one* of the following aspects of a holistic view of human beings: the indivisible body and mind, the limbic system, or character armor. Explain how this information is useful for the practice of massage therapy.

CHAPTER 4 CLINICAL APPLICATIONS OF MASSAGE

1. Clinical massage therapy describes applications of massage
   a. to improve athletic performance.
   b. to improve cardiovascular function.
   c. to treat a variety of pathologies.
   d. to treat immune system pathologies.

2. The "evidence" in evidence-based therapies should be.
   a. verifiable and subjective.
   b. verifiable and objective.
   c. unverifiable and objective.
   d. repeatable and subjective.

3. Principle-based therapy does *not* use
   a. consideration of the condition being treated.
   b. therapeutic potential of different treatment methods.
   c. creation of comprehensive treatment plan.
   d. recipe-based treatment protocols.

4. Understanding the scientific method, locating research articles, and analyzing research studies are all skills of
   a. research literacy.
   b. research design.
   c. clinical literacy.
   d. principle-based therapy.

5. When massage helps alleviate a diagnosed condition or eases its symptoms, it is _____ for treatment.
   a. suggested
   b. prescribed
   c. indicated
   d. contraindicated

6. When massage is used to reduce symptoms and discomfort of a disease without affecting a cure, it is considered _____ care.
   a. palliative
   b. integrated
   c. clinical
   d. direct

7. Relaxing hypertonic muscles, healthy scar formation, and relieving constipation are _____ effects of massage.
   a. indirect palliative
   b. complementary
   c. direct therapeutic
   d. direct palliative

8. This massage technique is effective in the treatment of repetitive strain injuries (RSIs).
   a. flow-flowing effleurage
   b. deep transverse friction
   c. fast-paced petrissage
   d. specific fine vibration

9. Massage of what body region has been found to be effective in reducing anxiety of hospitalized patients?
   a. feet
   b. abdomen
   c. arms
   d. back

10. What massage specialization has been found effective in treating postmastectomy lymphedema?
   a. myofascial massage
   b. lymphatic drainage massage
   c. neuromuscular therapy
   d. polarity therapy

11. Treating edema in cases of chronic cardiac, kidney, or liver problems is
   a. a specialization.
   b. palliative care.
   c. contraindicated.
   d. indicated.

12. Which of the following is *not* a finding in studies on the effects of massage on children with asthma?
   a. decreased peak airflow
   b. decreased airway irritability
   c. increased chest expansion
   d. fewer asthma attacks

13. Massage has been found to _____ some of the negative side effects from radiation and chemotherapy in persons being treated for cancer.
   a. increase
   b. stabilize
   c. accelerate
   d. reduce

14. Because of the potential for metastasis (i.e., spreading the cancer), massage should be avoided
   a. altogether.
   b. where a tumor has recently been removed.
   c. around the body's lymph nodes.
   d. on the feet.

15. One of the important effects of massage on preterm infants is
   a. strength gain.
   b. skin moisture.
   c. weight gain.
   d. hand-eye coordination.

16. Lower cortisol levels in the blood is an objective measure indicating
   a. increased stress.
   b. reduced stress.
   c. increased anxiety.
   d. potential insomnia.

17. Massage is beneficial for people with medical conditions worsened by
   a. increased circulation.
   b. relaxation.

c. body awareness.

d. stress.

18. Anxiety reduction, improved body awareness, and the ability to receive pleasurable nonsexual touch are especially important effects of massage for this special population.

    a. preterm infants

    b. survivors of physical abuse

    c. athletes

    d. institutionalized elderly

19. Which massage technique description below best describes Therapeutic Touch?

    a. sliding on top of the skin

    b. compression of soft tissues with the palm

    c. sweeping hand movements a few inches above the skin

    d. percussive movements over heavily muscled areas

20. Forceful thrusting movements to realign skeletal structures should be applied by massage practitioners

    a. never.

    b. as needed.

    c. with doctor's permission.

    d. with the client's consent.

Short Answer and Essay Questions

21. Defend an *evidence-based* approach to massage therapy. What does it mean, and how do scientific studies benefit the work of massage practitioners?

22. Distinguish between a *recipe-based* and *principle-based* approach to massage therapy. Explain how research is best used in the principle-based approach.

23. Explain the three useful ways of thinking about the clinical benefits of massage therapy (i.e., complementary, palliative care or direct therapeutic effects). Give of an example of massage used in a clinical setting for each approach.

24. Describe how massage is used in the treatment of *one* of the following categories of pathologies: edema and lymphedema, respiratory pathologies, or cancer. Identify the effects of massage that are beneficial in the treatment of the disease, and cite research studies where applicable.

25. Describe the use of massage in the treatment of psychological disorders. Identify the effects of massage that are beneficial in the treatment of the disorder, and cite research studies where applicable.

CHAPTER 5 ENDANGERMENT SITES, CONTRAINDICATIONS, AND CAUTIONS

1. The most basic rule of contraindications for massage therapy is
   a. watch your pressure.
   b. do no harm.
   c. trust your instincts.
   d. take calculated risks.

2. The _____ of the neck is an endangerment site.
   a. posterior cervical muscle area
   b. suboccipital muscle area
   c. anterior triangle
   d. posterior quadrangle

3. Thrusting movements for "cracking" the back are
   a. generally therapeutic.
   b. indicated when requested.
   c. a massage therapy specialty.
   d. outside the scope of massage.

4. Avoid pressure on the _____ of the sternum.
   a. manubrium
   b. body
   c. xiphoid process
   d. coccyx

5. Which of the following areas is *not* an endangerment site?
   a. upper back
   b. anterior side of elbow
   c. posterior knee aka (popliteal area)
   d. inguinal area

6. Deep effleurage on the extremities should be performed
   a. horizontally.
   b. proximal to distal.
   c. distal to proximal.
   d. randomly.

7. If your client feels searing, shooting electrical sensations when you massage an area, you are hitting a
   a. bone.
   b. nerve.
   c. blood vessel.
   d. lymph vessel.

8. Conditions or situations that make receiving massage inadvisable because of the harm it might do are called
   a. pathologies.
   b. indications.
   c. contraindications.
   d. endangerment sites.

9. For _____ contraindications, avoid massage in the immediate area.
   a. regional
   b. general

c. focal

d. physiological

10. Identify which of the following conditions are *general* and which are *regional*. Circle the correct answer.

a. rheumatoid arthritis	regional	general
b. athlete's foot	regional	general
c. malignant melanoma	regional	general
d. fever	regional	general
e. bruising	regional	general
f. varicose veins	regional	general
g. edema due to cardiac disease	regional	general
h. skin rash	regional	general
i. nausea	regional	general
j. appendicitis	regional	general

11. Avoid _____ if the client is ticklish.

a. lotions with menthol

b. tapotement or percussion techniques

c. light superficial stroking

d. prone position

12. When a client's immune system is suppressed, be especially careful with

a. personal and environmental hygiene.

b. room lighting.

c. kneading techniques.

d. pressure used.

13. Swollen glands indicate general _____ and are a likely contraindication for massage.

a. weakness

b. high blood pressure

c. cardiac disease

d. infection

14. For which type of edema is massage *indicated*?

a. pitted edema indicating tissue fragility

b. edema associated with sprained ankle

c. edema due to deep vein thrombosis

d. edema caused by liver disease

15. If your client has osteoporosis or is in a high-risk category for the disease,

a. do not perform massage.

b. avoid effleurage on the limbs.

c. avoid heavy tapotement.

d. avoid kneading leg muscles.

16. If your client comes for massage and feels a little nauseous and has been running a slight fever,

a. do not perform massage.

b. limit techniques to circulatory massage.

c. avoid heavy tapotement.

d. limit techniques to effleurage and kneading.

17. If your client comes in for a scheduled massage and was in a car accident earlier in the day and is now complaining of severe neck pain,

a. use light pressure when massaging the neck.

b. work trigger points in the neck and shoulders.

    c. do not massage, but refer the client to a doctor for diagnosis.

    d. avoid neck and shoulder stretches.

18. If a client's medication is needed for condition stability (e.g., insulin-dependent diabetic),

    a. schedule the session for *after* the client's scheduled dosage.

    b. schedule the session for *before* the client's scheduled dosage.

    c. shorten the session.

    d. avoid heavy pressure techniques.

19. If your client is taking a drug that weakens tissue integrity (e.g., corticosteroids), you should avoid

    a. effleurage techniques.

    b. light vibration.

    c. nerve strokes.

    d. skin rolling and wringing.

20. If your client is taking a medication that masks pain, you should

    a. ask for frequent client feedback about pressure.

    b. rely less on client feedback and more on palpation and observation.

    c. shorten the session.

    d. use heavy pressure without worrying about causing pain.

Short Answer and Essay Questions

21. Draw the outline of a body, front and back. Shade in *and* label the major endangerment sites for massage.

22. List the seven general principles for safety around endangerment sites.

23. Give five examples of general contraindications for massage.

24. Give five examples of regional or local contraindications for massage.

25. Identify four major categories of medications that require caution when being taken by a recipient of massage. For each category, give one example of how a practitioner might respond (e.g., related to scheduling of sessions, session length, or selection of massage techniques).

CHAPTER 6 GENERAL PRINCIPLES FOR GIVING MASSAGE

1. Professional boundaries help maintain
   a. dual relationships.
   b. counter transference.
   c. appropriate roles.
   d. transference.

2. Two common mistakes in the therapeutic relationship are losing the distinction between personal and professional lives and
   a. avoiding dual relationships.
   b. going outside your area of expertise.
   c. maintaining confidentiality of client information.
   d. keeping a professional demeanor.

3. _____ happens when a client transfers positive or negative feelings from the past onto the massage practitioner or the therapeutic relationship.
   a. Dual relationship
   b. Sympathy
   c. Transference
   d. Countertransference

4. Which of the following statements about touch is *not* correct?
   a. Touch deprivation is a problem only in early life.
   b. Humans have an innate touch hunger.
   c. Touch is the primary mode of interaction in massage.
   d. Touch is our most social sense.

5. Prepare for massage by being aware of your intention to be
   a. anxious and distracted.
   b. apprehensive and focused.
   c. compassionate and seductive.
   d. caring and compassionate.

6. Which of the following statements about touch and communication is *most* correct?
   a. Touch is secondary to verbal communication in massage.
   b. Touch communicates many things about the practitioner to a sensitive recipient.
   c. Good verbal skills can make up for a practitioner's distractedness and lack of confidence during massage.
   d. Recipients of massage are usually distracted and unaware of the touch of the practitioner.

7. Which of the following statements about culture and touch is *most* correct?
   a. Men in all cultures have similar comfort levels with touch.
   b. Women in all cultures are open to touch similarly.
   c. The association of touch with sex is similar in all cultures.
   d. Comfort levels with touch vary with cultural background.

8. Touching which of the following areas would require explicit permission from the massage recipient?
   a. upper arm
   b. lower abdomen
   c. feet
   d. neck

9. The process of soliciting permission to touch an area is called
   a. informed consent.
   b. intervention model.
   c. HIPAA rules.
   d. touch protocol.

10. Problems related to gender (i.e., in cross-gender or same-gender massage) can be best minimized by
    a. informed consent.
    b. mutual consent.
    c. keeping professional boundaries.
    d. compassionate touch.

11. Sexualizing the therapeutic relationship in massage is
    a. acceptable with mutual consent.
    b. acceptable between consenting adults.
    c. dependent on the circumstances.
    d. never acceptable.

12. The Intervention Model is used if a client
    a. is experiencing pain.
    b. refuses consent to touch an area.
    c. sexualizes the massage.
    d. talks too much during massage.

13. The first step in the Seven Step Intervention Model is to
    a. evaluate the client's response.
    b. stop the session using assertive behavior.
    c. restate your professional boundaries.
    d. ask the client to clarify their behavior.

14. The final step in the Seven-Step Intervention Model is to
    a. continue or discontinue as appropriate.
    b. restate your professional boundaries.
    c. describe the behavior you are concerned about.
    d. document the situation.

15. A general rule is that social talking during massage should be
    a. kept to a minimum.
    b. limited to a client's psychological problems.
    c. confined to family concerns.
    d. focused on the practitioner's life.

16. Release of unexpressed emotions during massage (e.g., sighing or crying) is
    a. unheard of.
    b. to be discouraged.
    c. normal and understandable.
    d. abnormal and deviant.

17. The ethical principle of confidentiality is
    a. limited to a client's health history.
    b. based on a client's right to privacy.
    c. limited by practitioner's freedom of speech.
    d. based on personal freedoms.

18. The HIPAA Privacy Rule is a federal standard designed to
    a. establish the right of practitioners to share client information.
    b. allow health professionals to share client information as desired.
    c. protect the medical records of individuals.
    d. enhance the electronic sharing of client information.

19. Which of the following would *not* be acceptable under the HIPAA Privacy Rule?
    a. Patients/clients can obtain copies of medical records.
    b. Patients/clients give written consent for use of their information.
    c. Patients/clients ask for correction of mistakes in their record.
    d. Patient/client information available to all employees in a clinic.

20. A comfortable temperature for a massage room is around
    a. 68°F.
    b. 75°F.
    c. 82°F.
    d. 90°F.

21. Lighting in a massage room should ideally be
    a. soft and indirect.
    b. hard and direct.
    c. dark and sleep inducing.
    d. restricted to natural sunlight.

22. Which type of sound should be *avoided* in a massage environment?
    a. music for relaxation.
    b. fish tank bubbling.
    c. popular music.
    d. silence.

23. It is a breach of professional ethics to watch your client getting undressed for massage except when
    a. you are also good friends.
    b. your client asks you to stay.
    c. your client has a disability and needs help.
    d. you are in the middle of a conversation.

24. Which of the following topical substances is the best choice if you desire lubrication during the massage warming phase but want more friction later?
    a. liniment
    b. vegetable oil
    c. mineral oil
    d. lotion

25. Which of the following topical substances is the best choice for a circulatory massage emphasizing effleurage and petrissage techniques?
    a. liniment
    b. oil
    c. lotion
    d. none—Dry rubbing is best.

26. When positioning a client in the supine position, place bolsters under
    a. shoulders and ankles.
    b. ankles and neck.
    c. knees and neck.
    d. lower back and knees.

27. The most important consideration in positioning a client is
    a. using the proper protocol.
    b. the client's safety and comfort.
    c. access to body areas.
    d. a practitioner's preference.

28. Which of the following statements about draping is *not* correct?
    a. Genitals are covered at all times.
    b. Women's breasts are covered with a few special exceptions.
    c. Mutual consent is an acceptable reason to ignore draping guidelines.
    d. The purpose of draping is modesty, boundaries, and warmth.

29. Which of the following describes good hand mechanics during compression techniques?
    a. wrist hyperextended
    b. reinforcing hand placed over the bottom hand metacarpals
    c. wrist flexed
    d. reinforcing hand placed over the bottom hand wrist

30. Which of the following describes good hand mechanics during thumb pressure techniques?
    a. thumb and wrist joints in straight line
    b. thumb abducted
    c. wrist in slight adduction
    d. wrist in hyperextension

31. An example of *poor* body mechanics while applying massage techniques is
    a. bend at the knees to lower yourself.
    b. keep back and neck in alignment.
    c. bend your back to get closer to the receiver.
    d. use weight transfer to apply pressure.

32. Which of the following practices will likely lead to physical and mental strain?
    a. performing 30 massage sessions per week
    b. performing four one-hour sessions in a day
    c. taking 15-minute breaks between sessions
    d. taking 30-minute break per three consecutive sessions

33. Which of the following statements about the use of lubricants is *not* correct?
    a. Use the least amount of lubricant needed to get the job done.
    b. Too little lubricant can cause skin irritation.
    c. Extra lubricant is used for massage of the face.
    d. Keep the lubricant off of the recipient's hair.

34. Which of the following statements about the sequence of techniques during massage is *not* correct?
    a. Deep specific techniques should be preceded by superficial warming.
    b. Deep specific techniques should be applied first.
    c. Smooth transitions between techniques add to a pleasant feel.
    d. Effleurage is a good transition technique.

35. Practitioners who focus the use of their techniques on a small area or a particular anatomical structure are said to working with
    a. intuition.
    b. sensitivity.
    c. specificity.
    d. rhythmical skill.

36. Tissue damage can result from using too much _____ when applying techniques.
    a. rhythm
    b. pacing
    c. specificity
    d. pressure

37. The rhythm for a relaxing massage is generally described as
    a. uneven and fast paced.
    b. uneven with varied pace.
    c. even and slow paced.
    d. even and fast paced.

38. The skillful blending of performance elements comprises the _____ of massage.
    a. art
    b. science
    c. philosophy
    d. anatomy

Short Answer and Essay Questions

39. List at least five different ways to establish and maintain good professional boundaries with a client or patient.

40. Describe a situation for which informed consent is appropriate. Explain step-by-step how you would apply the informed consent protocol in this situation.

41. Describe a situation for which the intervention model should be used. Explain step-by-step how you would apply the intervention model in this situation.

42. Describe the important environmental factors to consider when setting up a massage space.

43. Discuss different topical substances used with massage, including their properties, and appropriate uses in massage applications.

44. Describe the elements of good body mechanics for massage practitioners when they are working at a massage table, both standing and sitting.

45. Identify the important performance elements of massage applications. Discuss how each element is varied for different effects.

CHAPTER 7 WESTERN MASSAGE TECHNIQUES

1–7. Match the seven Western massage technique categories with the correct description below.

_____ 1. effleurage
_____ 2. petrissage
_____ 3. friction
_____ 4. tapotement
_____ 5. vibration
_____ 6. touch without movement
_____ 7. joint movements

a. passive touch
b. rubbing surfaces together
c. slide over skin
d. kneading and compression
e. stretching and mobilizing
f. percussive movements
g. quivering or trembling motion

8. Which of the following best describes effleurage used for relaxation?
   a. slow smooth strokes using moderate pressure
   b. fast strokes with uneven rhythm
   c. slow strokes with heavy pressure
   d. fast strokes using moderate pressure

9. Which descriptor below best describes the action of skin rolling?
   a. kneading
   b. wringing
   c. squeezing
   d. lifting

10. Using excessive pressure when applying petrissage techniques can result in
    a. more effective milking of tissues.
    b. tissue damage and bruising.
    c. muscle relaxation.
    d. better local circulation.

11. The _rubdown_ performed historically after physical exercise and a steam bath consisted mainly of
    a. effleurage techniques.
    b. vibration techniques.
    c. superficial friction.
    d. deep friction.

12. When applying deep friction, the fingertips move
    a. with the skin.
    b. over the skin.
    c. under the skin.
    d. The fingertips do not move.

13. Deep transverse friction used in rehabilitation is sometimes also called
    a. superficial friction.
    b. circular friction.
    c. Mennell friction.
    d. Cyriax friction.

14. Which of the following is *not* a principle of deep transverse friction used in rehabilitation?
    a. It is Applied over the precise site of the lesion.
    b. Applying maximum pressure is essential.
    c. Tissue must be in appropriate tension.
    d. Six to twelve sessions of 20 minutes each on alternate days gives best results.

15. Which of following best describes skillful application of tapotement techniques?
    a. rapid, heavy, and rhythmic
    b. rapid, light, and rhythmic
    c. slow, light, and rhythmic
    d. slow, heavy percussion

16. To lighten the impact of tapotement techniques, let the hands
    a. be stiff.
    b. rest briefly on the skin.
    c. bounce off of the skin.
    d. skim the skin.

17. This technique is often used for stimulating digestive organs.
    a. fine vibration on the abdomen
    b. coarse vibration of the abdomen
    c. tapotement of the abdomen
    d. friction over the stomach

18. Which form of coarse vibration involves movement at a joint?
    a. shaking
    b. jostling
    c. stretching
    d. ischemic friction

19. Simply laying the hands lightly on the body is called
    a. ischemic compression.
    b. static friction.
    c. passive touch.
    d. casual touch.

20. Direct pressure with enough force to cause blanching is called
    a. ischemic compression.
    b. passive touch.
    c. fine vibration.
    d. passive compression .

Short Answer and Essay Questions

21. Name and describe the six soft tissue manipulation technique categories of Western massage. Give two examples of specific techniques from each category.

22. Explain the physiological effects of each of the six soft tissue manipulation technique categories, and describe how these techniques are used in a massage session.

CHAPTER 8 JOINT MOVEMENTS

1–4. Match the categories of joint movements with the correct descriptor.

_____ 1. free active movements
_____ 2. assisted movements
_____ 3. resisted movements
_____ 4. passive movements

a. recipient totally relaxed during movement
b. practitioner helps recipient complete the movement
c. recipient performs the movement without assistance
d. practitioner counteracts the recipient's movement

5. Within the context of massage therapy, _____ are free, loose, and passive movements performed within the normal range of joint motion.
a. mobilizing techniques
b. stretches
c. contract-relax-stretch
d. reciprocal inhibition

6. _____ are *not* within the scope of massage therapy.
a. Mobilizing techniques
b. Stretches
c. Adjustments
d. Resisted movements

7. Passive joint movements performed to the limit of a joint's range of motion, and used to elongate the soft tissues in the surrounding area, are called
a. adjustments.
b. mobilizing techniques.
c. assisted movements.
d. stretches.

8. Which of the following statements about the typical uses of joint movements in massage therapy is *not* correct?
a. Joint movements are used to increase range of motion.
b. Joint movements are used to improve immune system function.
c. Joint movements are used to improve body alignment.
d. Joint movements are used to increase kinesthetic awareness.

9. The degree of movement commonly found at a particular joint is called its
a. maximum potential.
b. reciprocal limit.
c. kinetic dimension.
d. range of motion.

10. Joint movements are contraindicated in areas with
a. muscle tension.
b. tissue scarring.
c. inflammation.
d. shortened tendons.

11. _____ refers to resistance felt as the limit of the stretch is approached.
a. Drag
b. End feel

c. Kinetic

d. Integration

12. In *static stretches*, these types of movements are *avoided*.
    a. holding at point of resistance
    b. gentle controlled movements
    c. sudden bouncing movements
    d. movement to point of resistance

13. In the _____ technique, the recipient is asked to contract the muscle to be stretched before the stretch is applied.
    a. static stretch
    b. contract-relax-stretch
    c. reciprocal inhibition
    d. passive stretch

14. In techniques using _____ , the recipient is asked to contract the antagonist of the muscle to be stretched before the stretch is applied.
    a. static stretch
    b. contract-relax-stretch
    c. reciprocal inhibition
    d. passive stretch

15. In coordinating a stretch with the recipient's breathing, the stretch should be applied as the recipient
    a. inhales.
    b. exhales.
    c. holds his or her breath.
    d. whistles.

16. Deliberate joint cracking is allowed within the context of massage
    a. when a recipient asks for it.
    b. when there is informed consent.
    c. never.
    d. only on the back.

17. Do the following before performing stretches on a body area.
    a. Perform percussion to loosen up the joint.
    b. Warm the soft tissues with massage.
    c. Apply ice pack for five minutes.
    d. Remind the recipient that "no pain, no gain."

18. Which of the following is the *least* important indicator of the limit of applying a stretch on an individual recipient?
    a. range of motion chart
    b. palpation of "end feel"
    c. recipient feedback
    d. palpation of tissue resistance to the stretch

Short Answer and Essay Questions

19. Identify six possible uses for joint movements during massage sessions.

20. Describe how you would apply a stretch to the hamstring muscles using *contract-relax-stretch* (CRS). Explain the recipient's position, your technique, and what you would say to the recipient as you lead him or her through the stretch (include the role of breathing).

21. Describe how you would apply a stretch to the hamstring muscles using *reciprocal inhibition*. Explain the recipient's position, your technique, and what you would say to the recipient as you lead him or her through the stretch (include the role of breathing).

CHAPTER 9 FULL-BODY WESTERN MASSAGE

1. Which of the following statements about full-body Western massage is *most* correct?
   a. It is limited mainly to effleurage and petrissage techniques.
   b. It is primarily for general relaxation.
   c. It includes both general health and therapeutic goals.
   d. It is performed in a prescribed routine.

2. What is the recommended direction to move around the table from region to region for full-body Western massage?
   a. clockwise
   b. counterclockwise
   c. random direction
   d. figure eight

3. If the recipient needs to be alert immediately after the massage session (e.g., driving back to work), it is best to end the session with him or her in the _____ position.
   a. prone
   b. supine
   c. side-lying
   d. face-down

4. Which of the following is the best choice for a transition technique?
   a. friction
   b. vibration
   c. petrissage
   d. effleurage

5. Which of the following best describe the goals of finishing techniques?
   a. reconnect, promote calm, and signal the end of the session
   b. improve circulation, warm the area, and relax muscles
   c. improve joint mobility, apply oil, and finish the region
   d. warm the area, stimulate, and specific techniques

6. Which of the following tends to disrupt a sense of continuity and flow in a full-body massage session?
   a. orderly sequence from region to region
   b. smooth transitions
   c. removing hands abruptly
   d. skillful draping

7. How is a full-body massage session lasting 30 minutes different from a session lasting 60 minutes? The 30-minute session is
   a. faster-paced with more specificity.
   b. faster-paced with less specificity.
   c. slower-paced with more specificity.
   d. unevenly paced with more attention to detail.

8. Which of the following statements about full-body massage routines is *least* correct?
   a. Practitioners develop their own routine ways of performing massage.
   b. Routines evolve with further training and experience.
   c. Routines are modified to meet recipient needs.
   d. Routines rarely change once established.

9. "Slower paced with fewer specific and stimulating techniques" best describes what type of massage?
   a. circulatory massage
   b. athletic massage
   c. general relaxation massage
   d. therapeutically specific massage

10. Practitioners who integrate various forms of massage and bodywork with Western massage are described as
    a. eccentric.
    b. eclectic.
    c. prolific.
    d. prosaic.

CHAPTER 10 REGIONAL APPLICATIONS

1. The social and emotional associations people have for different body regions are examples of their
   a. anatomical structure.
   b. common pathologies.
   c. human meaning.
   d. clinical meaning.

2. The _____ of different body regions reminds massage practitioners to consider the wholeness of the body when performing massage.
   a. isolation
   b. interconnectedness
   c. uniqueness
   d. segmentation

3. The muscles of expression in the face (e.g., for smiling, frowning, and wrinkling the forehead) are
   a. involuntary muscles.
   b. skeletal muscles.
   c. attached to face bones.
   d. embedded in cutaneous tissue.

4. Effleurage over the eyelids should be performed
   a. with very light pressure.
   b. with heavy pressure.
   c. with enough pressure to massage the eyeball underneath.
   d. never.

5. Which of the following techniques is *most* effective for massaging the scalp muscles?
   a. coarse vibration
   b. tapotement
   c. circular friction
   d. basic effleurage

6. A three-dimensional sense of different body regions is enhanced by knowledge of
   a. skeletal structures in the area.
   b. sites of muscle attachments.
   c. location of visceral organs.
   d. layers of muscles from superficial to deep.

7. Back massage to promote falling asleep and restful sleep consists mainly of
   a. long gliding strokes.
   b. light tapotement techniques.
   c. fine vibration.
   d. superficial friction.

8. More pressure can be applied to the heavy muscles of the buttocks with less strain on the practitioner by
   a. use of the fingertips to apply techniques.
   b. use of the thumb to apply techniques.
   c. use of the elbow and forearm to apply techniques.
   d. avoiding the area.

9. Which technique is safest for massage over the popliteal area?
   a. light effleurage with broad flat palm of the hand
   b. deep stripping with thumbs

c. direct pressure with the elbow

d. rapping tapotement

10. Which of the following is a dangerous movement when massaging the feet?
    a. effleurage with the thumb between metatarsals
    b. effleurage with the fist on the bottom of the foot
    c. popping the toes
    d. mobilizing metatarsals with scissoring motion

11. Which of the following statements about the amount of pressure to use for massage of heavily muscled areas is *most* correct? In areas with large muscles
    a. use as much pressure as you can.
    b. use as much pressure as your client will allow.
    c. modify the amount of pressure according to condition of tissues.
    d. use your body weight to apply as much pressure as you can.

12. To impart vibration across the large shoulder muscles (i.e., upper trapezius), it is best to use
    a. fingertip vibration.
    b. an electronic vibrator.
    c. the elbow.
    d. knuckles of a loose fist.

13. Performance of breast massage requires
    a. a doctor's prescription.
    b. special training and informed consent.
    c. intuition and common sense.
    d. legal release.

14. The general direction of abdominal massage is
    a. medial to lateral.
    b. distal to proximal.
    c. counterclockwise.
    d. clockwise.

15. Which of the following techniques is commonly used to stimulate digestion and elimination during abdominal massage?
    a. fine vibration
    b. coarse vibration
    c. cupping tapotement
    d. kneading petrissage

Short Answer and Essay Questions

16. Explain important aspects of the human meaning for *one* of the following body regions: head and face, neck, back, or feet.

17. Describe a thorough massage of the foot including soft tissue manipulations and joint movements.

18. Describe an abdominal massage specifying the direction of application as well as specific techniques.

19. Describe a therapeutic sequence for the neck. Include soft tissue manipulation as well as joint movements.

20. Describe a therapeutic sequence for the lower back. Include soft tissue manipulation as well as joint movements.

CHAPTER 11 HYDROTHERAPY / THERMAL THERAPIES

1. Archeologists excavating the ancient ruins of the Mayan Civilization in Mexico and Central America (250–850 C.E.) have found
   a. massage tables.
   b. swimming pools.
   c. sweat baths.
   d. saunas.

2. This Austro-Hungarian farmer developed an entire system of baths, compresses, and other thermal therapies between 1829 and 1849.
   a. Hippocrates
   b. Vincent Priessnitz
   c. Pehr Ling
   d. J. Harvey Kellogg

3. This famous water cure advocate became the foremost authority on water-based therapies with his little book *My Water Cure* published in 1889.
   a. Sebastian Kneipp
   b. Pehr Ling
   c. Sir John Floyer
   d. Alain-Yvan Belanger

4. Bath (c. 1740), Harrogate (c. 1824), and Buxton (c. 1858) are examples of English
   a. Turkish baths.
   b. sweat baths.
   c. mineral water hospitals.
   d. Vichy showers.

5. Thermo-therapy involves hydrotherapy methods that are
   a. above normal body temperature.
   b. at normal body temperature.
   c. below normal body temperature.
   d. above freezing.

6. The recommended water temperature range for a relaxation whirlpool bath is
   a. 80° to 90°F (27° to 32°C).
   b. 95° to 105°F (35° to 41°C).
   c. 110° to 120°F (43° to 49°C).
   d. 130° to 140°F (54° to 60°C).

7. A type of shower in which shower heads surround the bather at different levels from head to toe is called the
   a. Kneipp shower.
   b. Vichy shower.
   c. Roman shower.
   d. Swiss shower.

8. The humidity in a steam room is at
   a. 50%.
   b. 75%.
   c. 100%.
   d. 125%.

9. The steam room can be an effective treatment for
   a. heart or circulatory problems.
   b. respiratory congestion.
   c. infection.
   d. skin rashes.

10. Which of the following is *not* associated with a sauna?
    a. dry heat
    b. wooden benches
    c. cold plunge
    d. whirling water

11. People who are weak or over 60 years old should limit their time in hot baths and steam to
    a. 15 minutes.
    b. 30 minutes.
    c. 45 minutes.
    d. 60 minutes.

12. Symptoms of having stayed in hot water or steam too long include
    a. lightheaded, nauseous, and headache.
    b. relaxed and flushed.
    c. chills and shivering.
    d. sweating.

13. Which of the following practices is recommended for safe use of thermo-hydrotherapy facilities?
    a. Eat just before using the facilities to avoid nausea.
    b. Drink a glass of wine to begin relaxation.
    c. Drink plenty of water to replace loss through sweating.
    d. Go barefoot in the facility to get maximum benefit from the heat.

14. Which of the following should you instruct your client to do before entering hydrotherapy facilities after massage?
    a. Eat a snack.
    b. Apply lotion.
    c. Wait 30 minutes.
    d. Exercise.

15. What type of hot packs are more penetrating for therapeutic applications?
    a. dry-heat packs
    b. moist-heat packs
    c. body-heat packs
    d. thermo-heat packs

16. A good place on your own body to check how hot a pack feels on the skin is the
    a. fingertips.
    b. outside elbow.
    c. inside wrist.
    d. knee.

17. What is typically used as a buffer between a moist-heat pack and the skin of the recipient to prevent burning?
    a. paper towels
    b. cloth towels
    c. pillow cases
    d. nothing

18. The maximum time for hot pack application on a local area is about
    a. 40 minutes.
    b. 30 minutes.
    c. 20 minutes.
    d. 10 minutes.

19. The third stage of sensation to expect with ice applications is
    a. numbness.
    b. cold.
    c. aching or burning.
    d. tingling or itching.

20. Ice massage is typically performed
    a. in a linear motion over a large area for about 20 minutes.
    b. in a circular motion over a small area for about 10 minutes.
    c. in a linear motion over a small area for about 30 minutes.
    d. in a spiral motion for about 20 minutes.

Short Answer and Essay Questions

21. Explain how you would integrate the use of hot packs with a full-body relaxation massage. Include the purpose, time of application, and safety precautions.

22. How would you instruct a client to use the hydrotherapy facilities of the spa or health club during his or her visit there for a massage session? Include the timing relative to the massage, the amount of time to stay in them, and other safety precautions. Limit to two different types of facilities.

CHAPTER 12 MYOFASCIAL MASSAGE

1. Limited mobility and postural distortions are two results of
   a. pliable fascia.
   b. fascial sheaths.
   c. fascial restrictions.
   d. collagen fibers.

2. Myofascial massage gained recognition in the United States in the 1970s as the result of the pioneering work of
   a. Pehr H. Ling
   b. Ida Rolf
   c. Elizabeth Dicke
   d. Johann Mezger

3. The three primary elements of fascia are
   a. ground substance, collagen, and elastin.
   b. muscle, gel, and elastin.
   c. fround substance, muscle, and lymph.
   d. tendons, ligaments, and sheaths.

4. Fascia becomes more pliable with the application of
   a. cold and compaction.
   b. cold and movement.
   c. heat and stretching.
   d. heat and compaction.

5. Fascia has a property called _____, by which it can change from a more liquid gel consistency to a more solid one, and vice versa.
   a. metabolism
   b. thixotropy
   c. respiration
   d. thickopathy

6. Fascial sheets are formed by _____ between collagen fibers.
   a. mechanical links
   b. fascial adhesions
   c. hydrogen bonds
   d. retinaculae

7. Anatomical fascial structures do *not* include
   a. body straps.
   b. visceral organs.
   c. retinaculae.
   d. fascial sheaths.

8. The quality of application of myofascial massage techniques can be described as
   a. fast and firm.
   b. slow and gentle.
   c. slow and compressing.
   d. fast and deep.

9. When myofascial tissues release, it feels like
   a. sharp break in adhesions.
   b. hardening of tissue.

c. melting or giving in tissues.
d. restriction in tissues.

10. Myofascial techniques are applied
    a. horizontally.
    b. vertically.
    c. perpendicularly.
    d. circularly.

Short Answer and Essay Questions

11. Name and describe the three different types of fascia distinguished as being at different depths in the body.
12. Identify and explain four functions of fascia in the body.
13. Explain the metaphor of fascia as a knitted sweater.
14. Explain how myofascial techniques release adhesions and result in more pliable tissues.
15. Describe four important guidelines for performing myofascial massage.

CHAPTER 13 NEUROMUSCULAR THERAPY

1. The doctor who pioneered trigger point therapy in the 1960s and who relieved muscular pain of a famous U.S. President with the method is
   a. Stanley Lief.
   b. Janet Travell.
   c. Bonnie Prudden.
   d. Johann Mezger.

2. Two essential criteria for identifying trigger points are
   a. redness and heat.
   b. soft spot and pain with pressure.
   c. redness and taut band.
   d. tender spot and taut band.

3. Always tender, prevents full lengthening, weakens the muscle, and refers pain on direct compression describes
   a. an active trigger point.
   b. a latent trigger point.
   c. a satellite trigger point.
   d. a deactiviated trigger point.

4. Trigger points that are only painful when pressed are called
   a. active.
   b. latent.
   c. deactivated.
   d. phantom.

5. An active trigger point radiates pain into its
   a. center.
   b. tender spot.
   c. zone of reference.
   d. nerve attachments.

6. Muscles in the immediate area of a trigger point often feel like
   a. rope.
   b. pudding.
   c. hills.
   d. valleys.

7. Ischemic compression techniques cause tissue blanching, followed by
   a. vasoconstriction.
   b. more blanching.
   c. reactive hyperemia.
   d. numbness.

8. The recommended amount of time to apply ischemic compression to a trigger point is
   a. 5–10 seconds.
   b. 20–60 seconds.
   c. two minutes.
   d. four minutes.

9. Good hand mechanics when applying ischemic compression with the thumb include
   a. thumb and wrist joints in straight alignment.
   b. thumb abducted.

   c. 90-degree angle between thumb and hand.

   d. wrist flexed and thumb abducted.

10. To complete the deactivation of a trigger point, the muscle affected should always be

   a. compressed.

   b. pinched.

   c. stretched.

   d. soaked.

Short Answer and Essay Questions

11. Give six examples of autonomic phenomena that can be "triggered" by active trigger points.

12. Discuss how trigger points are activated. Include both direct and indirect stimuli.

13. Describe methods of locating trigger points on a client/patient.

14. Describe in detail the method of deactivating a trigger point (TrP) using ischemic compression. Include point location, application of pressure, knowing when the point has released, and finishing.

15. Identify at least three different manual methods of deactivating a trigger point besides ischemic compression.

CHAPTER 14 LYMPHATIC DRAINAGE MASSAGE

1. Pioneers in the development of lymphatic drainage massage in Europe in the 1930s were
   a. Michael and Ethel Foldi.
   b. Emil and Astid Vodder.
   c. Pehr Ling and Johann Mezger.
   d. Eunice Ingham and Fred Stoffel.

2. What percent of the body's interstitial fluid is returned to the cardiovascular system by the lymph vessels?
   a. 1%
   b. 10%
   c. 20%
   d. 30%

3. What percent of the lymph vessels are located in the skin?
   a. 10%
   b. 30%
   c. 50%
   d. 70%

4. What feature of the lymph capillaries (i.e., initial lymphatics) is most affected by the application of lymphatic massage techniques?
   a. one-cell-thick walls
   b. cell membrane
   c. cell nucleus
   d. overflaps of cell junctions

5. The head, neck, chest, abdomen, and groin are the location of major clusters of
   a. lymphatic ducts.
   b. lymphangions.
   c. lymph nodes.
   d. precollector vessels.

6. The direction of application of lymphatic drainage massage techniques is determined by the
   a. location of the heart.
   b. deep collector vessels.
   c. superficial lymph drainage pathways.
   d. muscular contour.

7. Which of the following is a contraindication for lymphatic drainage massage?
   a. lymphedema
   b. malignant tumor
   c. allergy symptoms
   d. colitis

8. The pressure used for LDM techniques is best described as
   a. very light with only enough pressure to move superficial skin.
   b. moderate with enough pressure to engage muscle tissue.
   c. heavy with enough pressure to move fluid through deep vessels.
   d. fluctuating—sometimes light, sometimes heavy.

9. The direction of the active part of LDM techniques is best described as
   a. away from the targeted lymph nodes.
   b. away from the heart.

c. toward the targeted lymph nodes.
d. toward the deep lymph vessels.

10. Which of the following is *not* a correct principle of lymphatic drainage massage?
    a. Techniques are repeated 6–8 times in each spot.
    b. The area proximal to a node is treated before the area distal to the node.
    c. The skin should appear red after LDM.
    d. LDM techniques should not be painful.

Short Answer and Essay Questions

11. Draw a diagram of the initial lymphatics (i.e., lymph capillaries) and label important parts of the structure. Explain how lymphatic drainage massage techniques facilitate the flow of lymph fluid into these tiny vessels.

12. Draw an outline of a person and indicate (and label) major lymph node locations. Using arrows to indicate direction draw the pattern of lymph movement toward the thoracic and right lymphatic ducts (label location of ducts).

13. Explain the importance of pressure, direction, rhythm, and sequence when applying lymphatic drainage techniques.

14. Describe in detail one of the lymphatic drainage massage techniques.

CHAPTER 15 FOOT REFLEXOLOGY

1. In Zone Therapy, the body is imagined as being divided into 10 _____ zones with endpoints in the _____.
   a. transverse; ears
   b. diagonal; hands
   c. longitudinal; feet
   d. latitudinal; feet

2. Modern foot reflexology was developed by _____ in the 1930–1940s.
   a. Ida Rolf
   b. Eunice Ingham
   c. Mary McMillan
   d. Randolph Stone

3. Modern foot reflexology combines the theory of Zone Therapy with
   a. vibration of the sole of the foot.
   b. joint movements in the toes.
   c. effleurage of the tops and bottoms of the feet.
   d. compression and direct pressure to the feet.

4. One of major principles of Zone Therapy is that pressure applied anywhere in a zone affects the _____ zone.
   a. entire
   b. adjacent
   c. bottom of the
   d. corresponding

5. To relieve pressure on the recipient's knees, and to bring the feet to the proper height for the practitioner's good body mechanics, a bolster should be placed _____.
   a. behind the recipient's lower back.
   b. under the ankles.
   c. under the knees.
   d. behind the neck.

6. The following foot reflexology technique is used to apply pressure quickly and efficiently to spots on the bottom and sides of the feet.
   a. effleurage
   b. tapotement
   c. finger skipping
   d. thumb walking

7. The following foot reflexology technique is used to effectively apply pressure to the top of the foot.
   a. finger walking
   b. thumb walking
   c. finger skipping
   d. squeezing

8. The following foot reflexology technique is used to apply pressure to the toes.
   a. finger walking
   b. thumb walking
   c. twisting
   d. squeezing

9. The hook and backup technique is used to apply _____ pressure to spots on the bottom of the foot.
   a. light
   b. deep
   c. oscillating
   d. gliding

10. Which of the following statements best describes how the body's organs are shown on a reflexology map?
   a. Both feet have identical pictures of all of the body's organs.
   b. The right foot depicts organs found in the upper part of the body, and the left foot depicts those on the bottom part of the body.
   c. The right foot depicts organs found on the right side of the body, and the left foot depicts those on the left side of the body.
   d. The right foot depicts organs found on the left side of the body, and the left foot depicts those on the right side of the body.

Short Answer and Essay Questions

11. Explain how the theory of Zone Therapy relates to the reflexology maps of the feet.

12. Draw outlines of right and left foot bottoms. Be sure to draw the toes clearly to distinguish between the two feet. Draw in and label the following body structures in their correct locations on the feet according to the theory of reflexology: lung, sinuses, shoulders, heart, liver, stomach, kidney, and large intestine.

CHAPTER 16 POLARITY THERAPY

1. Polarity Therapy was developed by _____ in the early twentieth century.
   a. Eunice Ingham
   b. Mary McMillan
   c. Randolph Stone
   d. Toru Namikoshi

2. The original theory of Polarity Therapy was heavily influenced by
   a. European folk remedies.
   b. Ayurvedic medicine from India.
   c. Western medicine from Europe.
   d. Mayan healing practices from Central America.

3. The aim of Polarity Therapy is to remove obstructions to
   a. the free flow of energy.
   b. the circulatory system.
   c. the intestinal tract.
   d. lymph flow.

4. Comprehensive treatment with Polarity Therapy would include hands-on techniques and also
   a. acupuncture.
   b. exercise and nutrition.
   c. hydrotherapy.
   d. crystal energy balancing.

5. Polarity Therapy practitioners assess the health of an area primarily through
   a. written reports from clients.
   b. X-rays.
   c. tingling in their hands.
   d. visual inspection.

6. The principle of "love" in Polarity Therapy refers to
   a. sympathy for the client.
   b. attitude of surrender and openness.
   c. sentimental caring.
   d. affectionate touch.

7. Polarity Therapy is a gentle art, and nothing is ever
   a. rhythmic.
   b. repeated.
   c. forced.
   d. felt.

8. Which of the following best describes Polarity Therapy techniques?
   a. tapping, shaking, and gliding
   b. sliding, thorough kneading, and vibrating
   c. holding, gentle rocking, and pressing
   d. direct pressure to acupoints

9. The "tummy rock" technique in Polarity Therapy is best described as
   a. rocking the abdomen gently while resting the other hand on the forehead.
   b. abdominal massage using a rocking petrissage.
   c. making the fist like a rock and compressing the abdomen.
   d. rock solid vibration of the abdominal area.

10. A good finishing technique for a Polarity Therapy session is
    a. outside ankle press.
    b. inside ankle press.
    c. forearm stimulation.
    d. brushing off.

Short Answer and Essay Questions

11. Describe some of the objective changes that have been observed in recipients of Polarity Therapy that indicate that the session is having a physiological effect.

12. Discuss the concept of *energy* in the context of Polarity Therapy. Describe what a Polarity Therapy practitioner feels as an indication of energy movement or obstruction.

CHAPTER 17 ASIAN BODYWORK THERAPY THEORY

1. The scope of practice of Asian Bodywork Therapy includes the assessment and treatment of
   a. physiological pathologies according to Western science.
   b. energetic imbalances according to Western science.
   c. musculoskeletal imbalances according to Chinese medicine.
   d. energetic imbalances according to Chinese medicine.

2. The earliest known text on Chinese medicine is
   a. *Red Emperor's Classic of Chinese Folk Remedies.*
   b. *Yellow Emperor's Classic of Chinese Medicine.*
   c. *The Book of Changes.*
   d. *The Little Red Book of China.*

3. Traditional Asian Medicine arrived in Japan as *kampo,* the Chinese way, in about
   a. 500 B.C.E.
   b. 100 C.E.
   c. 600 C.E.
   d. 1600 C.E.

4. Which if the following is *not* a principle of the theory of Traditional Asian Medicine?
   a. The universe is dynamic, moving, changing.
   b. Humans are related and connected to all that exists.
   c. Theory is based on what can be reliably measured, predicted, and controlled.
   d. Humans are an integral part of the universe.

5–8. Identify the following descriptions as associated with Yin or Yang. Select "Yin" or "Yang" for each question.

_____ 5. light and energetic

_____ 6. warm and expanding

_____ 7. deep and cool

_____ 8. dense and contracting

9. Which of the following describe Yang aspects of the body?
   a. exterior and lateral aspects of the limbs
   b. interior and medial aspects of the limbs
   c. organs that store essences extracted from food
   d. front of the body

10. The Chinese character for Qi depicts
    a. rice cooking in a pot with steam escaping.
    b. winds and waves.
    c. the sunny side of a hill.
    d. trees and raindrops.

11. Extracting the essential nutrients from food and air is an example of which of the following functions of Qi?
    a. transporting
    b. protecting
    c. transforming
    d. warming

12. What are the Five Elements of Chinese medicine?
    a. earth, air, fire, water, and rock
    b. water, air, earth, clay, and metal
    c. metal, wind, water, fire, and wood
    d. water, wood, fire, earth, and metal

13. What is the most Yin of the Five Elements?
    a. earth
    b. water
    c. fire
    d. metal

14. Which of the following is a good example of the Sheng Cycle, also called the creation or generating cycle?
    a. Metal, such as an ax, cuts Wood.
    b. Earth channels Water.
    c. Wood feeds Fire.
    d. Water extinguishes Fire.

15. Which of the following is a good example of the Ko Cycle, also called the controlling or acting cycle?
    a. Fire makes ash which becomes Earth.
    b. Fire melts Metal.
    c. Water nourishes Wood (e.g., trees).
    d. Metals are carried in Water that springs out of the Earth.

16. Which of the following statements about energy channels is *most* correct?
    a. Channels are external energy pathways all located just under the skin.
    b. Channels follow the circulatory system and are located alongside of blood vessels.
    c. Channels are energy pathways both external and internal (i.e., deep).
    d. Channels are energy pathways that follow the nervous system and parallel the spinal nerves.

17. According to the Chinese Body Clock, the energy channels flow through the body in a natural
    a. rhythmic daily cycle.
    b. rhythmic weekly cycle.
    c. unpredictable daily pattern.
    d. rhythmic cycle that varies seasonally.

18. The traditional Four Pillars of Assessment are
    a. blood test, eye exam, palpation, and health history.
    b. strength, flexibility, agility, and speed.
    c. looking, touching, listening/smelling, and asking.
    d. blood pressure, pulse, deep breathing, and skin exam.

19. How many classical pressure points are located along the major energy channels?
    a. 58
    b. 150
    c. 365
    d. 655

20. Which of the following statements about acupoints is *not* correct?
    a. Acupoints are places where Qi can collect.
    b. Acupoints are best used to address specific symptoms.
    c. Acupoints can be influenced by applying pressure.
    d. Acupoints are used for treatment of energy imbalances.

Short Answer and Essay Questions

21. Contrast traditional Chinese medicine with Western scientific medicine. How does each view the body? How does each view an individual's place in the universe? How does each view the nature of health and disease?

22. Draw the Yin/Yang symbol, and explain its meaning. Identify the nature of Yin and Yang and the five principles of interaction between them.

23. Name and describe the five functions of Qi.

24. Explain the proper use of acupoints in Asian bodywork therapy.

CHAPTER 18 AMMA—TRADITIONAL JAPANESE MASSAGE

1. The Chinese characters pronounced *anmo*, or *amma* in Japanese, mean
   a. to heal with massage.
   b. to health by kneading.
   c. to calm by rubbing.
   d. to rejuvenate by touching.

2. In the Edo Period in Japan (1603–1857 C.E.) amma became an occupation for
   a. the elderly.
   b. the blind.
   c. the lame.
   d. widows.

3. Traditional amma was introduced in the United States in 1971 by Takashi Nakamura, who trained amma practitioners for the
   a. Kabuki Hot Springs in San Francisco.
   b. Canyon Ranch in Tucson.
   c. Melzer's Spa in Hot Springs Arkansas.
   d. Saratoga Springs in New York.

4. Amma sessions are performed
   a. with oil or lotion.
   b. with special Japanese oil.
   c. with sesame oil.
   d. without oil or lotion.

5. What is the first question in the five question screening process for amma?
   a. Have you had any recent injuries?
   b. Are you on any medications?
   c. Have you ever had a massage before?
   d. Are you allergic to any oils?

6. What is the best way to ensure that the receiver is always comfortable during the session?
   a. Use very little pressure to apply techniques.
   b. Tell them that amma is healthy and to be open to it.
   c. Give them permission to give feedback about their comfort.
   d. Screen beforehand to eliminate the fainthearted.

7. In performing amma techniques, pressure is applied most efficiently by using
   a. arm and shoulder strength.
   b. weight transfer.
   c. hand and shoulder strength.
   d. special hand tools.

8. Perpendicularity is a principle of amma technique application to make sure that
   a. hands and fingers are protected.
   b. pressure is off of the wrist.
   c. pressure is applied at a 45-degree angle to the acupoint.
   d. pressure is sinking straight into the acupoint.

9. The shoulder in line with the elbow, the wrist, and the thumb joints is an example of which principle of body mechanics?
   a. stacking the joints
   b. perpendicularity

c. weight transfer
d. kata

10. Which of the following statements about the use of kata for learning a form like traditional Japanese massage is *not* correct?
    a. Kata allows practice of skilled touch with confidence.
    b. Kata as developed by a master is proven effective.
    c. Kata provides the opportunity to experiment with different ideas.
    d. It is the kata that teaches the student massage.

CHAPTER 19 ZEN SHIATSU—AN OVERVIEW

1. In the Japanese language, *shiatsu* means
   a. gentle pressure.
   b. finger pressure.
   c. finger action.
   d. pressure on points.

2. Which of the following best describes Zen Shiatsu?
   a. It views body from an anatomical structural perspective.
   b. It uses the same meridians and tsubos as acupuncture.
   c. Harder pressure is applied at acupoints than in other shiatsu forms.
   d. It uses broader set of meridians and lighter pressure than other shiatsu forms.

3. According to Traditional Asian Bodywork theory, both the cause and effect of good health is
   a. balanced flow of ki in meridians.
   b. obstructed flow of ki in meridians.
   c. proper musculoskeletal alignment.
   d. proper digestion and elimination.

4–8. Match the following body functions with their associated meridians [Table 19-1].

   _____ 4. intake of ki
   _____ 5. interpretation of the emotional environment
   _____ 6. purification
   _____ 7. intake of food
   _____ 8. circulation

   a. stomach
   b. heart
   c. heart constrictor
   d. lung
   e. bladder

9. According to the concept of *homeostasis*, whenever an external force is applied to a dynamic system, at least one change must occur in the system to establish
   a. a continuing system of imbalance.
   b. a permanent condition of stability.
   c. a new condition of balance.
   d. a switch to static or nondynamic system.

10. Ki or life energy that has a high vibrational quality feels
    a. light, fast, and heated.
    b. light, slow, and cold.
    c. heavy, fast, and heated.
    d. heavy, fast, and cold.

11. The quality of ki called *kyo* refers to
    a. hot ki.
    b. deficient ki.
    c. excessive ki.
    d. flowing ki.

12. The quality of ki called *jitsu* refers to
    a. deficient ki.
    b. excessive ki.

c. balanced ki.
d. heavy, slow ki.

13. Most energy imbalances can be traced to _____ of ki that retards a meridian's function.
    a. an excess
    b. an absence
    c. a strengthening
    d. a high vibrational

14. Diagnostic areas for each of the 12 meridians are found on the
    a. arms.
    b. chest.
    c. abdomen.
    d. feet.

15. Which of the following best describes the effective application of Zen Shiatsu techniques?
    a. rigid hand with focus on moving receiver's ki
    b. rigid hand with focus on angle of pressing tsubos
    c. relaxed hand with focus on receiver's ki as source of healing
    d. relaxed hand with intention to force ki to flow freely

16. In the Japanese language, the word *tsubo* means
    a. sunny hill.
    b. vase.
    c. vortex of energy.
    d. force of life.

17. Which of the following results from using weight transfer rather than pure muscular strength to apply firm pressure to tsubos?
    a. The receiver does not participate in the healing process.
    b. The practitioner dominates the process of healing.
    c. The practitioner's sensitivity is lessened.
    d. It draws the receiver's own energy into the area being touched.

18. Which type of rhythm is used to apply pressure to a jitsu meridian to assist in the redistribution of excess ki?
    a. waltz rhythm
    b. slow rhythm
    c. fast rhythm
    d. varying, slow then fast

CHAPTER 20 JIN SHIN DO®

1. Jin Shin Do can be translated as the Way of the
   a. Great Healer.
   b. Gentle Warrior.
   c. Compassionate Spirit.
   d. Finger Pressure.

2. Environmental, social, emotional, and physical tension and stress held in the musculature is called
   a. feathering.
   b. armoring.
   c. local points.
   d. key points.

3. In Jin Shin Do, channels that collect energy from other meridians that have excess energy are called
   a. governing vessels.
   b. collection channels.
   c. prime meridians.
   d. strange flows.

4. Assessment of meridians in Jin Shin Do is performed by determining which specific points on the_____ are tense or sore.
   a. arm
   b. back
   c. abdomen
   d. chest

5. Which of the following most accurately describes the basic Jin Shin Do pressure technique?
   a. A distal point is held for about two minutes while local points are pressed.
   b. Three or four acupoints are held simultaneously for about two minutes.
   c. A local point is held for about two minutes while distal points are pressed one after the other.
   d. One point at a time is pressed for about two minutes each along the affected meridian.

6. In Jin Shin Do, the usual procedure is to release body segments from
   a. the top down.
   b. the bottom up.
   c. left to right.
   d. right to left.

7. The pressure used on points in Jin Shin Do is best described as
   a. light but not so light as to tickle.
   b. light but enough to move the skin.
   c. medium and almost painful.
   d. firm but not so deep that the receiver cannot relax.

8. In Jin Shin Do, the point most needing release is called the
   a. top point.
   b. local point.
   c. distal point.
   d. segment point.

9. Which of the following is *not* a sign that a point has released?
   a. The finger sinks deeper into the tissues.
   b. The muscle contracts against the pressure.
   c. A pulse or increase in pulsation is felt.
   d. The recipient feels decrease in sensitivity at the point.

10. In the Jin Shin Do back release, the local point is
    a. on the top of the head.
    b. at the sacrum.
    c. between the eyes (third eye).
    d. in the lower back.

CHAPTER 21 SPORTS AND FITNESS

1. Sports massage as practiced in North America is based on
   a. traditional Chinese medicine.
   b. lymphatic drainage massage.
   c. traditional Western massage.
   d. Ayurvedic massage.

2–6. Match the five major applications of sports massage with the correct description.

   _____ 2. recovery
   _____ 3. remedial
   _____ 4. rehabilitation
   _____ 5. maintenance
   _____ 6. event

   a. to improve a debilitating condition
   b. to help prepare for and recover from a specific competition
   c. an all-purpose massage received regularly to address the athlete's needs
   d. to facilitate healing after a disabling injury
   e. addresses sore, stiff muscles and overall fatigue from strenuous exertion

7. A technique commonly used in sports massage to increase circulation and warm up the muscles when an athlete is clothed is
   a. static friction.
   b. tapping tapotement.
   c. rhythmic compression.
   d. fine vibration.

8. Which of the following best describes a typical pre-event massage session?
   a. 30-minute session, soothing, and medium pace
   b. 15-minute session, relaxing, and slow pace
   c. 15-minute session, stimulating, and faster pace
   d. 30-minute session, relaxing, and remedial applications

9. Which type of sports massage session combines recovery with remedial applications of massage?
   a. maintenance
   b. rehabilitation
   c. pre-event
   d. postevent

10. Which of the following best describes a typical postevent massage soon after the event?
    a. 45-minute duration, stimulating, and faster-paced
    b. 30-minute duration, heavy, and faster-paced
    c. 15-minute duration, light, and fast-paced
    d. 15-minute duration, light, and slower-paced

Short Answer Essay Questions

11. Distinguish between maintenance, remedial, and rehabilitation sports massage using examples for clarification.

12. Name forms of hydrotherapy typically available in gyms and health clubs. Describe how different forms of hydrotherapy can be used to enhance the effects of recovery massage.

13. Describe in detail the application of pre-event sports massage including goals of the session, duration, types of massage techniques used, and other important factors.

14. Describe in detail the application of postevent sports massage including goals of the session, duration, types of massage techniques used, and other important factors.

15. Choose a specific sport or fitness activity (e.g., running, swimming, tennis, baseball, golf, bowling, soccer, bicycling) for this exercise. Describe how the nature of the sport would affect your plan for maintenance massage of an athlete who participates in the activity regularly.

CHAPTER 22 MOTHER AND CHILD

1. Which of the following is *not* a characteristic of a typical pregnancy posture?
   a. head forward
   b. belly out
   c. knees slightly bent
   d. feet turned out

2. Which of the following is contraindicated in pregnancy massage?
   a. massage of the lower back
   b. abdominal massage
   c. foot massage
   d. shoulder massage

3. Which of the following is *not* a contraindication for massage of a pregnant woman?
   a. nausea
   b. fever
   c. vaginal discharge
   d. lower back pain

4. The massage room should be kept _____ for the comfort of most pregnant women.
   a. warmer
   b. cooler
   c. more stimulating
   d. lighter

5. Usually when massaging a pregnant woman, your table height should be set
   a. lower than usual.
   b. higher than usual.
   c. same as usual.
   d. on lowest setting.

6. Which of the following statements about positioning for a pregnant woman is *not* correct?
   a. For the first few months, many women can lie prone comfortably.
   b. Lying flat on the back is safe at all stages of pregnancy.
   c. Bolsters can be used to prop the recipient into a reclining position.
   d. Side-lying is the most common position for pregnancy massage.

7. In which of the following areas should deep massage be avoided in advanced stages of pregnancy?
   a. upper back and shoulders
   b. inner thighs
   c. feet
   d. inside upper arms

8. Which of the following best describe the qualities of a typical pregnancy massage?
   a. stimulating and fast-paced
   b. upbeat and deep
   c. gentle and relaxing
   d. vigorous and specific

9. During pregnancy, a woman's connective tissues naturally soften to facilitate delivery. What significance does that have for massage practitioners performing pregnancy massage?
   a. It causes some instability in joints and so joint movements should be performed gently and carefully.
   b. It loosens ligaments in the shoulders and so massage of upper arms should be avoided.
   c. It causes swelling in the arms and hands and so massage in that area should be vigorous and deep.
   d. It stretches ligaments in the feet, so foot massage should be avoided in later stages of pregnancy.

10. Which of the following techniques can be performed safely on the abdomen of a pregnant woman?
    a. vibration
    b. undulating petrissage
    c. nerve strokes
    d. none of the above

11. Which of the following is *not* an appropriate goal of infant massage?
    a. relieving trigger points
    b. improving sleep
    c. aiding digestion and elimination
    d. learning to relax

12. The most important contribution of massage to the overall healthy development of infants is that it
    a. improves circulation
    b. aids digestion
    c. provides tactile and kinesthetic stimulation
    d. calms babies

13. Which of the following statements about infant massage is *not* correct?
    a. Infant massage is simple, gentle, yet firm in application.
    b. Infant massage should not be given to preterm infants.
    c. Infant massage helps calm colicky babies.
    d. Massaging her infant promotes milk production in the mother.

14. Which of the following would you *avoid* when performing infant massage?
    a. playful interaction
    b. eye contact with the infant
    c. talking or singing during massage
    d. deep pressure on the tissues

15. In addition to abdominal massage, which of the following infant massage techniques helps promote bowel movements when repeated several times?
    a. gentle squeeze and twist of the legs
    b. arm movement across the chest (hug) and then out to the sides
    c. leg movement bringing knees to chest and then straightening
    d. long stroke over the back and legs with infant prone

Short Answer Essay Questions

16. Describe the typical pregnancy posture, and identify the stresses it creates on the body. Explain how this affects the goals for pregnancy massage.

17. List at least five potential benefits of pregnancy massage.

18. Describe how you would set up an ideal environment for pregnancy massage. List at least five factors that you would take into consideration.

19. Identify at least five contraindications or cautions for pregnancy massage.

20. Describe the four major possibilities for positioning a pregnant recipient for massage. Discuss when you would use each one, and when you would avoid it.

CHAPTER 23 HEALTHY AGING

1. Which of the following is *not* a common physical effect of aging?
   a. slower nerve conduction
   b. thinner dryer skin
   c. increase in bone mass
   d. less efficient immune system

2. At what age do the first signs of aging typically appear?
   a. 30
   b. 40
   c. 50
   d. 60

3. Which of the following statements about the elderly is *not* correct?
   a. Elders have an accumulated lifetime of diseases and injuries.
   b. Elders are more likely to have chronic health problems.
   c. Elders are more likely to be on medication.
   d. Elders are more similar to each other than any other age group.

4. Which physiological age category of elders would you treat like a typical middle-aged adult when giving massage?
   a. frail
   b. age appropriate
   c. robust
   d. institutionalized

5. What is the best way to help frail elders change position or sit up after massage?
   a. Cradle their bodies as you help them.
   b. Pull them by their arms at the elbow into a sitting position.
   c. Grab their hands and pull to desired position.
   d. Just lift their heads as they attempt to sit up.

6. What is the suggested length of time for the first massage session with a frail elder?
   a. no time limit
   b. 15–20 minutes
   c. 35–40 minutes
   d. 55–60 minutes

7. Which position is typically the most uncomfortable for elders to stay in for long periods of time (e.g., over 20 minutes)?
   a. supine
   b. prone
   c. reclining
   d. side-lying

8. What caution should be taken with clients who have had joint replacements?
   a. Avoid all joint movements.
   b. Perform joint movements as with normal client.
   c. Perform extra joint movements, especially stretches to the limit.
   d. Limit joint movements to those approved by the client's health care provider.

9. The best way to prevent bruises and tears in the thin, delicate skin of the elderly is to
   a. use moderate pressure when applying vigorous friction to dry skin.
   b. stop if you see bruising or bleeding.

c. use gentle pressure and sufficient lubricant.

d. watch recipient's face for signs of pain and then lighten pressure.

10. Which area of the neck can usually be massaged safely in elderly recipients?

a. anterior

b. lateral

c. posterior

d. none of the above

Short Answer Essay Questions

11. List eight common physical effects of aging.

12. Explain the special benefits of massage for the elderly population.

13. Summarize the findings of research on the benefits of massage for the institutionalized elderly.

14. Name the three physiological age categories for the elderly, and describe characteristics of people in each category. Explain massage considerations for each category.

15. List at least five goals for massage for healthy aging, and describe the techniques appropriate for achieving each goal.

CHAPTER 24 TERMINALLY ILL AND DYING

1. Palliative care refers to
   a. care that results in the cure of a disease.
   b. last efforts to cure a terminal disease.
   c. relieving the symptoms of a disease without effecting a cure.
   d. integrative health care in searching for a cure for a disease.

2. Programs designed specifically to provide for the needs of the terminally ill near the ends of their lives are referred to as _____ programs.
   a. hospital
   b. hospice
   c. nursing home
   d. lying-in hospital

3. For those who are unable to speak, or are withdrawn, the touch of massage offers a unique opportunity for _____ communication.
   a. verbal
   b. nonverbal
   c. psychic
   d. telepathic

4. In Farnslow's description of her use of Therapeutic Touch with the dying, she says that she places her hand _____ to offer a sense of peace and calm to the recipient.
   a. on the feet of the person
   b. on the abdomen
   c. on or near the shoulder
   d. over or near the heart

5. The *most* correct description of massage techniques used with the terminally ill and dying is
   a. specific and direct.
   b. pointed and firm.
   c. simple and gentle.
   d. complex and focused.

6. Which of the following is *not* a realistic benefit for family and other nonprofessional caregivers who give massage to their terminally ill loved one?
   a. sense of accomplishment in helping to cure the loved one
   b. something active to do with the loved one
   c. sense of connection with loved one
   d. provides mutual comfort for giver and loved one

7. Key attitudes for massage practitioners working with the terminally ill and dying are that they be
   a. objective, distant, clinical.
   b. caring, supportive, accepting.
   c. judgmental, sympathetic, closed.
   d. clinical, judgmental, careful.

8. The *most* correct description of the duration of massage for the terminally ill or dying is
   a. short—as short as 10–20 minutes of contact.
   b. the same as is standard massage—60 minutes.
   c. long—The longer the better.
   d. long—As long as the facility will allow.

9. Which of the following is the best area to massage for getting to know new patients, and for non-professional caregivers and volunteers?
   a. head and shoulders
   b. feet and legs
   c. hands and arms
   d. chest and abdomen

10. Working through feelings about illness, death, and dying with a friend, coworker, or supervisor is part of
    a. physical self-care.
    b. emotional self-care.
    c. therapeutic protocol.
    d. clinical approach.

Short Answer Essay Questions

11. List the most important physical, emotional, and social benefits of massage for the terminally ill and dying.

12. Explain how in the wellness model, someone who is terminally ill can be said to be striving for high-level wellness despite that fact that he or she is going to die soon.

13. Describe the qualities and techniques of massage for sessions with the terminally ill and dying.

14. List the benefits of hand and arm massage for the terminally ill and dying. Describe the qualities and techniques of the massage.

15. Describe a holistic self-care strategy when working with the terminally ill and dying.

CHAPTER 25 SEATED MASSAGE IN THE WORKPLACE

1. The modern massage chair was invented in the
   a. 1920s.
   b. 1940s.
   c. 1960s.
   d. 1980s.

2. Which of the following was *not* part of the original concept for the massage chair?
   a. to make massage more accessible to the general public
   b. able to be transported easily
   c. to be used for Western massage with application of oil or lotion
   d. to be able to receive massage sitting up

3. Which of the following statements about the benefits of seated massage in the workplace is *not* correct?
   a. helps prevent repetitive strain injuries
   b. reduces mental alertness and makes workers sleepy
   c. reduces stress levels of employees
   d. relieves tension headaches

4. The most common duration for seated massage in the workplace is
   a. 5–10 minutes.
   b. 15–20 minutes.
   c. 25–30 minutes.
   d. 55–60 minutes.

5. Which of the following techniques is *not* appropriate for giving massage over clothing?
   a. friction.
   b. kneading.
   c. compression.
   d. deep effleurage.

6. Light tapotement to the head has the effect of
   a. putting the recipient to sleep.
   b. stimulating and increasing mental alertness.
   c. general relaxation.
   d. improved circulation.

Short Answer Essay Questions

7. Explain the popularity of workplace massage. Identify at least four important factors.

8. Summarize the benefits of massage both to the individual worker and to the employer.

9. Give an example of a worker who could benefit from workplace massage. Describe his or her job, work station, and specific benefits of massage for his or her situation.

10. Describe a seated massage session for the workplace. Include the duration, the goals, the techniques used, and the general sequence of the routine.

Test Bank Answer Key

CHAPTER 1 HEALING MASSAGE—A WELLNESS PERSPECTIVE

1. c
2. d
3. b
4. a
5. a
6. d
7. b
8. c
9. d
10. b
11. a
12. b
13. d
14. b
15. c
16. b
17. d
18. e
19. a
20. f
21. c
22. a
23. d
24. b
25. b

26. Explain the difference between the concepts of *healing* and *curing*. Why is the concept of *healing* a better fit for the natural healing arts and philosophy?

   Sample Answer: The connotation of *curing* is of an *outside force* given to a *passive recipient/patient*, while *healing* implies the existence of an *innate force* at work from within and the recipient is an *active participant* in his or her own recovery. The concept of an innate healing force is basic to the natural healing philosophy.

27. Name and describe the four major massage and bodywork traditions. Give examples of each.

   Sample Answer: The four major massage and bodywork traditions are (1) native and folk, (2) Ayurvedic, (3) Asian bodywork therapy, and (4) Western massage. *Native and folk traditions* are passed down through the generations within families or by tribal and village healers and are based on what has been done in the past and on experience. Examples are Hawaiian lomi-lomi and Hispanic healers called curanderas. The *Ayurvedic tradition* originated in India and can be traced to ancient texts called the Vedas. Different types of oils are chosen carefully for each recipient of Ayurvedic massage. *Asian bodywork tradition* is based in Chinese medicine including theory of qi, energy channels, and acupoints. Forms of ABT include amma, acupressure, and shiatsu. The *Western massage tradition* is based on Western anatomy and physiology and includes the seven basic technique categories. Forms of Western massage include the classic Swedish massage, and contemporary forms like myofascial massage and lymphatic drainage massage.

28. Name and describe the seven basic Western massage technique categories. Give an example of a specific massage technique for each category.

   Sample Answer: The seven basic Western massage technique categories are (1) *effleurage* (i.e., sliding and gliding movements), (2) *petrissage* (i.e., kneading, lifting, and wringing movements), (3) *friction* (i.e., rubbing two surfaces together as in superficial and deep friction), (4) *tapotement* (i.e., percussion movements), (5) *vibration* (i.e., oscillating, quivering, or trembling movements), (6) *touch without movement,* such as passive touch or holding, and (7) *joint movements,* such as mobilizing techniques and stretches.

29. Discuss the relationship between conventional Western medicine and therapies that are called *alternative* and *complementary*. Explain the concept of *integrative health care* and how it differs from that of *CAM* therapies. Use examples from massage therapy in your discussion.

   Sample Answer: Conventional Western medicine (CWM) is the mainstream or regular medical practice in Western areas such as North America and Europe and is now practiced all over the globe. Methods of healing that are different from conventional Western medicine and used instead of CWM are called *alternative* therapies (for example, the use of an Asian bodywork therapy such as shiatsu instead of CWM). *Complementary* therapies are used in conjunction with CWM but are secondary CWM treatment (for example, relaxation massage used in palliative care of a hospitalized patient). Complementary and alternative medicine (CAM) is always seen in contrast to CWM. In *integrative health care* settings, a wide variety of healing methods, including CWM and CAM therapies, are viewed on more equal terms with the best methods chosen for an individual case. For example, a patient with colitis may be prescribed regular massage to reduce stress along with medication and a change in diet and exercise.

30. Draw the Wellness Pyramid, labeling the levels from bottom to top. Use the Wellness Pyramid to explain the many different reasons people seek massage. Be specific in your examples.

   Sample Answer: See Figure 1–5 for the Wellness Massage Pyramid. Starting with the base of pyramid and moving toward the top, someone might receive massage to *treat* a stress related illness like colitis; or in *recovery* from surgery to form a healthy scar; or to *prevent* a repetitive strain injury like tennis elbow; or to *maintain health* through relaxation and good circulation;

or for *personal growth* by better connecting the mind and body; or for *enjoyment of life* through the pleasures of healing touch.

CHAPTER 2 HISTORY OF MASSAGE

1. c
2. a
3. d
4. a
5. c
6. b
7. a
8. c
9. b
10. c
11. a
12. c
13. b
14. d
15. b
16. c
17. c
18. a
19. b
20. d
21. Describe the uses of massage in the ancient civilizations of China, India, Greece, and Rome. Give approximate dates (e.g., circa 500 B.C.E.) and one or two examples of how massage was used in each society.

Sample Answer: In *ancient China,* the basic philosophy of Chinese medicine was described in the *Yellow Emperor's Classic of Chinese Medicine* (c. 500 B.C.E.). Finger pressure was applied to acupuncture points and a form of massage called tuina was developed to balance energy or qi in the body.

Ayurvedic medicine in *ancient India* goes back to at least 500 B.C.E. and is based on ancient scriptures called the Vedas. Massage with oils is used to balance the life force or *prana* in energy centers called *charkas.*

In *ancient Greece* (c. 400–300 B.C.E.) massage was used by physicians such as Hippocrates for healing illness and injuries and in the gymnasia to prepare athletes for physical activity and help them recover after exercise.

In *ancient Rome* (c. 200 B.C.E.–400 C.E.) massage was used by physicians to prevent and treat certain diseases and in the Roman baths along with exercise, steam rooms, and hot and cold pools as a wellness measure.

22. Trace the early development of Western massage and the contributions of Pehr H. Ling and Johann Mezger. Include approximate dates and terminology used at the time.

Sample Answer: *Pehr H. Ling* (1776–1839) of Sweden developed a system of alternative medicine called *medical gymnastics* that used active and passive movements to treat chronic diseases. He founded a school in Stockholm in 1813 that trained medical gymnasts and took in students from all over the world. His system spread to many countries in North America and Europe and was known in English speaking countries as the Swedish Movement Cure. The passive movements in his system included joint movements and massage-like movements that he called by descriptive terms like *shaking, pressing, stroking,* and *pinching.*

Johann Mezger (1838–1909), a physician in Amsterdam, categorized soft tissue manipulation into four broad technique categories using the French terms *effleurage, petrissage, tapotement,* and *friction.* Mezger's success in healing certain ailments helped massage gain acceptance in medical circles in the late nineteenth century.

Many practitioners used techniques from both the Swedish movement cure and massage in treatments, and the combination eventually evolved into what was known as Swedish massage by the early twentieth century.

23. Discuss the development of massage in the early twentieth century as used in physical therapy. Include important people and their contributions and approximate dates.

Sample Answer: During World War I (c. 1914–1918) courses in *reconstruction* were developed to teach the use of massage and the Swedish movements for rehabilitation of wounded soldiers. Also influential was the work of Sir Robert Jones, an orthopedic surgeon from England, and James B. Mennell, who worked with Jones at the Special Military Surgical Hospital in England in the early twentieth century. Mennell stressed the importance of care and gentleness in performing massage. Mary McMillan, also associated with Jones' clinic in England in the early twentieth century, became the chief aide at Walter Reed Army Hospital in the United States and instructor for *reconstruction aides,* who worked in military hospital rehabilitation and massage units. McMillan was the director of physiotherapy at Harvard Medical School from 1921 to 1925, when she wrote a popular physical therapy text *Massage and Exercise.* The profession of physical therapy continued to evolve as those trained initially in rehabilitation of war wounds applied physiotherapy to other areas like industrial injuries and treating victims of polio.

24. Discuss the natural healing movement of the late nineteenth and early twentieth centuries. Trace its origin, philosophy, people, institutions, and the types and uses of massage within that context.

Sample Answer: Conventional medicine, which relied increasingly on new developments in drugs and surgery, became more main stream in the late nineteenth century. At that time, a countermovement arose based on traditional natural health and healing methods such as herbs, good nutrition, exercise, fresh air and sunshine, vegetarianism, laughter, hydrotherapy, and massage. The natural healing philosophy includes the belief that living beings have innate healing powers that are best assisted by various natural methods.

A leading proponent of "biologic living" was J. Harvey Kellogg (1852–1943), director of the Battle Creek Sanitarium, a famous health resort in Michigan. Massage was provided at the Sanitarium to help improve digestion and circulation and for relaxation. Bernarr Macfadden (1868–1955) spearheaded a movement called *physical culture,* which popularized the natural healing philosophy in the early twentieth century through books, *Physical Culture* magazine, a radio show, and health resorts. Macfadden developed a system of massage and movements that he called physcultapathy.

25. Describe the revival of interest in massage in the 1970s. Include the contributions of the counterculture, human potential movement, the Esalen Institute, and the wellness movement.

Sample Answer: There were several cultural changes and movements that occurred in the 1970s that resulted in the revival of interest in massage. For example, the *counterculture* or "hippie" movement, in rebelling against the conservative 1950s, sought ways to reconnect with the emotional, spiritual, and sensual aspects of their lives, and explored massage as a way of getting better in touch with their whole selves. The *human potential movement*, closely identified with the Esalen Institute in Big Sur, California, explored ways of reaching the limits of human potential. Different forms of massage and bodywork, movement practices such as tai chi and qi gong, meditation, psychotherapy in "encounter groups" and a variety of other practices were taught at Esalen. A form of massage emphasizing its sensual nature was developed at Esalen and became popular in the 1970s.

In addition, the *wellness movement* started among health and fitness professionals in the 1970s. The wellness movement redefined health as more than the absence of disease to include leading a vibrant meaningful life in all its dimensions (i.e., physical, mental, emotional, and spiritual). It promoted many of the practices of the old natural healing philosophy emphasizing self-responsibility for health through proper diet, exercise, stress reduction, massage, and so on. All of these factors combined led to a heightened awareness of and interest in massage in the 1970s that continues to this day.

26. Discuss the professionalization of massage in the 1990s. Include the major milestones.

Sample Answer: In the 1990s, the evolution of massage into a mainstream health profession reached several milestones. The Office of Alternative Medicine (OAM) was established at the National Institutes of Health in 1992, and acknowledged massage as an important "unconventional medical practice." The number of research studies on the efficacy of massage increased, and the first research center for massage and touch therapies was established in 1992 (i.e., the Touch Research Institute at the University of Miami). The AMTA Foundation was founded in 1992 to fund research projects and disseminate information on massage research. A national credential for massage practitioners was first available in 1992 (i.e., National Certification for Therapeutic Massage and Bodywork). Educational standards for massage programs were developed by the Commission on Massage Therapy Accreditation, which received United States Department of Education (USDE) recognition in 2002. Finally several surveys done in the 1990s showed that consumers were seeking complementary therapies, including massage, in increasing numbers.

CHAPTER 3 EFFECTS AND BENEFITS OF MASSAGE

1. b
2. a
3. c
4. d
5. c
6. a
7. c
8. b
9. a
10. b
11. d

12. a

13. b

14. c

15. b

16. d

17. a

18. c

19. d

20. a

21. b

22. b

23. a

24. d

25. c

26. Explain the three phases of the process of tissue repair. Discuss the uses of massage to facilitate the process including contraindications, and goals and specific techniques appropriate for each phase.

> Sample Answer: The three phases of tissue repair are *inflammation* to stabilize the injured area, *regeneration* to restore tissue structure, and *remodeling* for healthy scar formation. Massage is contraindicated in the immediate location of the injury during the inflammation phase. During the regeneration phase, circulatory massage helps remove debris from the site and brings in building materials for tissue restoration. During the remodeling phase, deep transverse friction is used for healthy scar formation.

27. Explain four different ways that massage is used to elicit muscle relaxation. Include description of specific massage techniques.

> Sample Answer: First, relaxation massage using effleurage and petrissage stimulates the parasympathetic nervous system, which generally reduces muscle tension. Second, there may be a conscious letting go of general muscle tension as the recipient assumes a passive state during massage. Third, application of a variety of massage techniques increases sensory stimulation, which causes normalization of reflex pathways of hypertonic muscles resulting in their relaxation. Fourth, a technique called *muscle approximation* can be used on a specific muscle or muscle group to reduce muscle tone. In this technique, the practitioner slowly and forcibly draws the attachments of the muscle closer together, which decreases stretch on the muscle spindles resulting in muscle relaxation.

28. Discuss the contributions of massage to the healthy functioning of *one* of the following body systems: cardiovascular, lymphatic, integumentary.

> Sample Answer: Massage contributes to the healthy functioning of the *cardiovascular system* in a number of ways. First, massage is known to increase local circulation through mechanical action of techniques, such as effleurage and petrissage, and reflex effects of capillary vessel dilation. Deep effleurage performed from distal to proximal enhances venous return in the limbs. General massage has a temporary effect of lowering blood pressure and, with regular relaxation massage, a more long-term effect of blood pressure reduction due to stimulation of the parasympathetic nervous system. Massage also increases the number of red blood cells in circulation.

29. Explain the use of massage for wellness, related to *one* of the following organism-level phenomena: growth and development, pain, stress. Describe specific massage techniques where applicable.

Sample Answer: Studies show that massage promotes proper growth and development of infants. The caring touch provided by massage stimulates tactile nerve endings in the skin, which helps the developing infant's nervous system organize its circuitry. The arm and leg movements stimulate the kinesthetic nerves, which also influences proper organization of reflexes deep within the nervous system. Pleasurable tactile experiences such as massage early in life are associated with the development of desirable personality traits such as calmness, gentleness, and nonaggression.

30. Explain the benefits of massage for psychological well-being. Include at least three specific effects and massage forms or techniques where applicable.

Sample Answer: Massage promotes psychological well-being by improving mental clarity, reducing anxiety, providing for release of unexpressed emotions held in the body, and increasing feelings of well-being. Stimulating massage techniques such as tapotement and fast-paced performance of technique combinations stimulate the nervous system and improve mental clarity. Relaxation massage quiets the nervous system and reduces anxiety. Relaxation massage is also known to release endorphins, which increases general feelings of well-being.

31. Name and describe five mechanisms used to explain how the effects of massage are produced. Give an example of each mechanism.

Sample Answer: The effects of massage can be explained by five different mechanisms. First, *mechanical effects* are the result of physical forces such as compression, stretching, and vibration of tissues (e.g., breaking adhesions with deep transverse friction). Second, *physiological effects* occur at the cellular, tissue, and organ system levels (e.g., eliciting the relaxation response through stimulation of the parasympathetic nervous system). Third, *reflex effects* are functional changes mediated by the nervous system (e.g., pain reduction). Fourth, *body-mind effects* that involve the connection of mind, body, and emotions (i.e., anxiety reduction through relaxation massage). Fifth, *energetic effects* where the body's energy flow is improved and obstructions are removed.

32. Discuss *one* of the following aspects of a holistic view of human beings: the indivisible body and mind, the limbic system, or character armor. Explain how this information is useful for the practice of massage therapy.

Sample Answer: *Character armor* is the concept that suppressed emotions can be held in the body as muscle tension. It is a good example of the body-mind connection. For example, unexpressed anger can be held in the muscles that would be used to strike out, or unexpressed grief can be held in the muscles of the chest or neck. Knowledge of the potential causes of muscle tension can help the massage practitioner better plan a session to achieve relaxation and understand the potential for release of emotions during massage.

CHAPTER 4 CLINICAL APPLICATIONS OF MASSAGE

1. c
2. b
3. d
4. a

5. c

6. a

7. c

8. b

9. d

10. b

11. c

12. a

13. d

14. b

15. c

16. b

17. d

18. b

19. c

20. a

21. Defend an *evidence-based* approach to massage therapy. What does it mean, and how do scientific studies benefit the work of massage practitioners?

Sample Answer: An *evidence-based approach* to massage therapy means that applications of massage are based on objective and verifiable research studies. This approach offers an advantage in an integrative health care system. Research studies can also substantiate the benefits of massage for certain pathologies and help identify contraindications. Research can also help massage practitioners apply techniques better to achieve session goals.

22. Distinguish between a *recipe-based* and *principle-based* approach to massage therapy. Explain how research is best used in the principle-based approach.

Sample Answer: In *recipe-based* massage a recipient receives exactly the same treatment or application of techniques as others with the same condition, while in *principle-based* massage the practitioner chooses massage techniques to achieve session goals for each client and his or her unique situation. Therefore, the massage is different even for clients with similar conditions. Research is used in principle-based massage to help the massage therapist decide on the best plan for treatment.

23. Explain the three useful ways of thinking about the clinical benefits of massage therapy (i.e., complementary, palliative care, direct therapeutic effects). Give an example of massage used in a clinical setting for each approach.

Sample Answer: *Complementary* massage enhances a primary treatment method (e.g., by creating a more favorable environment for healing, as in improving immune system function). *Palliative care* reduces symptoms and discomfort without affecting a cure (e.g., in reducing anxiety of hospitalized patients). *Direct therapeutic effects* directly treat the problem condition (e.g., relieving constipation with abdominal massage).

24. Describe how massage is used in the treatment of *one* of the following categories of pathologies: edema and lymphedema, respiratory pathologies, or cancer. Identify the effects of massage that are beneficial in the treatment of the disease, and cite research studies where applicable.

Sample Answer: Lymphatic drainage massage is used in the *treatment of edema* caused by musculoskeletal injuries. The mechanical action of lymphatic massage techniques moves lymph fluid from the area and back into circulation. This reduces swelling in the immediate site of the injury and helps prevent secondary injury to tissues.

25. Describe the use of massage in the treatment of psychological disorders. Identify the effects of massage that are beneficial in the treatment of the disorder, and cite research studies where applicable.

Sample Answer: Massage can reduce anxiety and increase feelings of well-being in patients being treated for psychological disorders. In one study, children and adolescents hospitalized for depression were given massage, which lessened their depression.

CHAPTER 5 ENDANGERMENT SITES, CONTRAINDICATIONS, CAUTIONS

1. b
2. c
3. d
4. c
5. a
6. c
7. b
8. c
9. a
10.
    a. regional
    b. regional
    c. general
    d. general
    e. regional
    f. regional
    g. general
    h. regional
    i. general
    j. general
11. c
12. a
13. d
14. b
15. c
16. a
17. c
18. a
19. d
20. b

21. Draw the outline of a body, front and back. Shade in *and* label the major endangerment sites for massage.
    See Figure 5-1.

22. List the seven general principles for safety around endangerment sites.
    1. Always adjust your pressure for the part of the body you are working on, the condition of the tissues, and the age of the person.
    2. Avoid heavy pressure over unprotected nerves, blood, and lymph vessels.
    3. Be careful around joints, where delicate structures are less protected.
    4. If you feel a pulse, it means you are on an artery. Move off of the spot.
    5. If the receiver feels searing, burning, shooting, or electrical sensations, it means you are on a nerve. Move off the spot.
    6. Proceed with caution around any abnormal structure.
    7. When in doubt, do not take a chance that might lead to injury.

23. Give five examples of general contraindications for massage.

    Sample Answer: Five examples of general contraindications for massage are (1) fever, (2) nausea, (3) appendicitis, (4) blood poisoning, (5) uncontrolled high blood pressure.

24. Give five examples of regional or local contraindications for massage.

    Sample Answer: Five examples of local or regional contraindications for massage are: (1) athlete's foot, (2) bruise, (3) varicose veins, (4) inflamed arthritic joints, (5) burns.

25. Identify four major categories of medications that require caution when being taken by a recipient of massage. For each category, give one example of how a practitioner might respond (e.g., related to scheduling of sessions, session length, and selection of massage techniques).

    Sample Answer: Four major categories of medications that require caution are those that (1) alter sensation, (2) affect blood and circulation, (3) compromise tissue integrity, or (4) alter mood. If a recipient's medication alters sensation of pain, then a practitioner should rely more on his or her own judgment and palpation skills to determine the appropriate amount of pressure to use. If a recipient is taking blood thinners, then a practitioner should use lighter pressure to prevent bruising. If a recipient is taking a corticosteroid, then the practitioner should avoid deep massage techniques and techniques with shearing or wringing action. If a recipient is taking medication that causes abnormal fatigue such as an antianxiety drug, the length of the session might be shortened.

CHAPTER 6 GENERAL PRINCIPLES FOR GIVING MASSAGE

1. c
2. b
3. c
4. a
5. d
6. b
7. d
8. b
9. a
10. c

11. d

12. c

13. b

14. d

15. a

16. c

17. b

18. c

19. d

20. b

21. a

22. c

23. c

24. d

25. b

26. c

27. b

28. c

29. b

30. a

31. c

32. a

33. c

34. b

35. c

36. d

37. c

38. a

39. List at least five different ways to establish and maintain good professional boundaries with a client or patient.

> Sample Answer: Five different ways to establish and maintain good professional boundaries are (1) proper draping, (2) professional clothing, (3) avoiding dual relationships, (4) respecting client's freedom of choice, (5) avoiding personal self-disclosure.

40. Describe a situation for which informed consent is appropriate. Explain step-by-step how you would apply the informed consent protocol in this situation.

> Sample Answer: Informed consent would be appropriate if you wanted to work into the muscle attachments high on the thigh of a runner. You would (1) explain that you would like to massage muscle attachments high on the thigh, (2) explain that it would help relax the thigh muscles and improve flexibility, (3) explain to the recipient that he or she will be securely draped and that you will be working muscle attachments, (4) ask permission to go ahead, (5)

create atmosphere where the client is free to refuse either before or during the proposed treatment.

41. Describe a situation for which the intervention model should be used. Explain step-by-step how you would apply the intervention model in this situation.

Sample Answer: The Intervention Model should be used when a client sexualizes the massage—for example, intentionally touches your thigh and makes a sexual remark. If this happened during the session, you would (1) stop the massage, (2) describe what happened ("You touched my leg and then made a sexual remark,"), (3) confirm ("Is that an accurate description of what just happened?"), (4) Clarify the client's response ("You admit that that was your intention"), (5) Assess the situation as inappropriate, (6) Decide to stop the massage and clarify that you do not perform sexual massage, (7) Document the session in the client file and in a separate incident report.

42. Describe the important environmental factors to consider when setting up a massage space.

Sample Answer: When setting up a massage space, the following factors should be considered: room temperature, air quality, lighting, sound, dressing arrangements, overall cleanliness, and neatness.

43. Discuss different topical substances used with massage, their properties, and appropriate uses in massage applications.

Sample Answer: Topical substances used with massage include *liniments,* which are watery substances that contain counterirritants such as camphor, menthol, and cayenne pepper. They are typically applied after massage of an area. *Oils* such as vegetable and mineral oils provide a slippery surface for massage and add moisture to the skin. Oils are used for massage that involves a lot of sliding over the skin. *Lotions* are semiliquid substances with moisturizing agents that are absorbed into the skin. Lotions are useful if sliding is desirable at the beginning of the massage and more friction desired after a while.

44. Describe the elements of good body mechanics for massage practitioners when they are working at a massage table, both standing and sitting.

Sample Answer: Good body mechanics involve keeping the body in good alignment. That means bending at the knees instead of the waist to lower the body, moving the whole body instead of just the arms to apply pressure, keeping wrists in a neutral position instead of hyperextended, and avoiding bending the back and neck. When standing at the massage table, use martial arts stances to lower the body from the knees, shifting weight to apply pressure. When sitting, keep feet flat on the floor and back straight.

45. Identify the important performance elements of massage applications. Discuss how each element is varied for different effects.

Sample Answer: Important performance elements of massage applications include sequence of techniques and routines, specificity and direction, pressure, rhythm, and pacing. Each element is varied to produce different effects (e.g., a relaxing massage is evenly paced and applied slowly with smooth transitions, using light to medium pressure). A stimulating massage would be fast paced with uneven rhythm and using stimulating techniques like vibration and tapotement. Massage with more specificity would be used to treat specific small area or individual structures, or conditions such as trigger points. Pressure generally starts out light and then deepens as the area is warmed and more specific techniques are applied, and lightens again as massage of the area is completed.

The general sequence of techniques for an area is opening and warming techniques, circulation and relaxation techniques, specific techniques such as friction in a specific structure, finishing techniques, and transition techniques.

CHAPTER 7 WESTERN MASSAGE TECHNIQUES

1. c
2. d
3. b
4. f
5. g
6. a
7. e
8. a
9. d
10. b
11. c
12. a
13. d
14. b
15. b
16. c
17. a
18. b
19. c
20. a

21. Name and describe the six soft tissue manipulation technique categories of Western massage. Give two examples of specific techniques from each category.

> Sample Answer: (1) *Effleurage* techniques slide or glide over the skin with smooth continuous motion (e.g., basic sliding effleurage and nerve strokes). (2) *Petrissage* techniques lift, wring, or squeeze soft tissues (e.g., basic two-handed kneading and compressions). (3) *Friction* techniques rub one surface over another repeatedly (e.g., superficial warming friction and deep cross-fiber friction). (4) *Tapotement* techniques are rapid percussive movements (e.g., hacking and cupping). (5) *Vibration* techniques cause oscillating, quivering, or trembling motion (e.g., fine vibration with fingertips and coarse vibration by shaking a muscle). (6) *Touch without movement* is defined by touch but no visible motion (e.g., passive touch and holding).

22. Explain the physiological effects of each of the six soft tissue manipulation technique categories, and describe how these techniques are used in a massage session.

> Sample Answer: (1) *Effleurage* stimulates touch receptors in the skin, activates the parasympathetic nervous system for relaxation, enhances circulation of fluids and venous return in the limbs, and can provide a passive stretch of tissues. Effleurage is used to apply oil or lotion, to begin a session, as a connecting and transition technique, and to conclude massage of an area. (2) *Petrissage* techniques "milk" tissues of metabolic waste products, increase local circulation, assist venous return, separate muscle fibers, and evoke muscle relaxation. Petrissage is used most often after an area is warmed with effleurage and before very specific techniques such as deep friction, with the exception of compressions that are sometimes used for initial warm-

ing when working without lubricant. (3) *Superficial friction* stimulates touch receptors in the skin, increases superficial circulation, and warms the skin, and it is used when warming is desired or when stimulating an area. *Deep friction* increases local circulation, separates tissues, and breaks adhesions, and is used after initial warming techniques to address specific structures such as tendons. (4) *Tapotement* provides nervous system stimulation and increases mental clarity. It is usually used as a finishing technique for a specific area or as a connecting technique when finishing one side of the body (i.e., front or back). (5) *Vibration* techniques stimulate the nervous system, provide sensory input, and can result in muscle relaxation. Fine vibration techniques are used in specific areas for the stimulating effects (e.g., on the abdomen). Coarse vibration is used to encourage muscle relaxation as when jostling the leg. (6) *Touch without movement* has a calming influence on the nervous system and is believed by some to help balance energy. It is typically used when finishing work on a specific area or when ending the entire massage session.

CHAPTER 8 JOINT MOVEMENTS

1. c
2. b
3. d
4. a
5. a
6. c
7. d
8. b
9. d
10. c
11. b
12. c
13. b
14. c
15. b
16. c
17. b
18. a

19. Identify six possible uses for joint movements during massage sessions.

> Sample Answer: Six uses for joint movements during massage sessions are (1) stretch surrounding soft tissues, (2) increase range of motion, (3) stimulate production of synovial fluid, (4) increase kinesthetic awareness, (5) stimulate muscle relaxation, (6) build muscle strength (resisted movements).

20. Describe how you would apply a stretch to the hamstring muscles using *contract-relax-stretch* (CRS). Explain the recipient's position, your technique and what you would say to the recipient as you lead him or her through the stretch (include the role of breathing).

> Sample Answer: For this hamstring stretch the recipient is lying supine, with their straight leg off of the table (flexed at the hip). I am facing the head of the table while holding the flexed leg with two hands. I will stretch the hamstrings by gently pushing the leg further into flex-

ion to its limit. Before I apply the stretch, I ask the recipient to push against my hands (extending the leg) with about 80% of his or her strength (to contract the hamstrings) and hold for about 10 seconds. Afterward, I say "relax," "take a deep breath," "slowly exhale." While the recipient is exhaling I apply the stretch.

21. Describe how you would apply a stretch to the hamstring muscles using *reciprocal inhibition*. Explain the recipient's position, your technique, and what you would say to the recipient as you lead him or her through the stretch (include the role of breathing).

    Sample Answer: For this hamstring stretch the recipient is lying supine, with their straight leg off of the table (flexed at the hip). I will stretch the hamstrings by gently pushing the leg further into flexion to its limit. Before I apply the stretch, I ask the recipient to push against my hands (flexing at the hip) with about 80% of his or her strength (to contract the quadriceps) and hold for about 10 seconds. I am standing so that I can apply resistance to his or her attempts to lift the leg with the quadriceps muscles. Afterward, I say "relax," "take a deep breath," "slowly exhale." While he or she is exhaling I apply the stretch.

CHAPTER 9 FULL-BODY WESTERN MASSAGE

1. c
2. a
3. b
4. d
5. a
6. c
7. b
8. d
9. c
10. b

CHAPTER 10 REGIONAL APPLICATIONS

1. c
2. b
3. d
4. a
5. c
6. d
7. a
8. c
9. a
10. c
11. c

12. b

13. b

14. d

15. a

16. Explain important aspects of the human meaning for *one* of the following body regions: head and face, neck, back, feet.

   Sample Answer: As we "face the world," much of our consciousness is focused on the head, which is center for thinking and processing information. The human meaning of the *head and face* is also related to all of the sensory organs located there (e.g., sight, smell, taste, and hearing). We communicate with others through structures of speech and with facial expression and take nourishment into our mouths. Emotional distress can be seen as tension in the face muscles.

17. Describe a thorough massage of the foot including soft tissue manipulations and joint movements.

   Sample Answer: A thorough massage of the foot would include both soft tissue and joint movement techniques. Begin by applying lubricant to the foot and ankle, warming the tissues. Mobilize the ankle using the heel of the hands, the metatarsals with a scissoring motion, and the toes with figure eights. Apply effleurage on the top of the foot with fingertips, and then on the foot bottom with a lightly closed fist. Press spots all along the foot bottom for improved energy flow and to stimulate other parts of the body according to reflexology theory. Finish with more effleurage and slapping the bottom of the foot with the back of the hand for pleasant stimulation.

18. Describe an abdominal massage specifying the direction of application as well as specific techniques.

   Sample Answer: Abdominal massage is performed in a clockwise direction. Start by applying lubricant to the area with effleurage moving clockwise. Follow with fingertip vibration in the same pattern. Apply gentle undulating compression of the area with the palm of the hand. Follow with circular effleurage, then horizontal stroking around the waist (between lower ribs and pelvis), and finish with passive touch with the palm of the hand on the belly.

19. Describe a therapeutic sequence for the neck. Include soft tissue manipulation as well as joint movements.

   Sample Answer: A therapeutic sequence for the neck might start with application of lubricant across the shoulders and up the posterior cervical muscles. (Avoid massage of the anterior triangle of the neck.) Use effleurage with fingertips, palms, or loose fist to warm the shoulder and cervical muscles. Deepen pressure as tissues relax and soften. Follow with circular friction along the posterior cervical muscles. Apply direct pressure with thumb or fingertips to the trapezius muscle and deeper cervical muscles. Reconnect the area with some deep effleurage. Apply some gentle stretches to the neck (e.g., flexion, horizontal flexion, rotation). Finish with effleurage to reconnect the area, and then end with holding the head gently in neutral position (face up).

20. Describe a therapeutic sequence for the lower back. Include soft tissue manipulation as well as joint movements.

   Sample Answer: A therapeutic sequence for the lower back might start with application of lubricant to the entire back with effleurage, followed by circular friction along the paraspinal muscles. Continue to warm lower back muscles with superficial friction with the knuckles. Once these muscles are thoroughly warmed, apply stripping to the muscles of the lower back along the spine between the rib cage and the pelvis. Follow with direct thumb pressure along the quadratus lumborum. Repeat stripping to the area. With fingers on one side of the spine and the thumb on the other side, gently rock the lower back from side to side to create movement in the spine. Finish with effleurage to reconnect the lower back to the entire back.

CHAPTER 11 HYDROTHERAPY/THERMAL THERAPY

1. c
2. b
3. a
4. c
5. a
6. b
7. d
8. c
9. b
10. d
11. a
12. a
13. c
14. c
15. b
16. c
17. b
18. c
19. c
20. b

21. Explain how you would integrate use of hot packs with a full-body relaxation massage. Include the purpose, time of application, and safety precautions.

Sample Answer: I would integrate the use of hot packs at the beginning of a relaxation massage with the recipient prone, placing the packs on the recipient's upper back and shoulders. The purpose would be to facilitate general relaxation, as well as warming and specific relaxation of the back muscles. I would check the recipient's health history to make sure there were no contraindications, do a visual check of the back for possible contraindications, and ask permission (informed consent) to use the hot packs. I would use layers of cloth towels to protect the skin from burning and ask to be notified if the packs get too hot. I would massage the legs while the hot packs were on the back. I would remove the hot packs after 15–20 minutes, and then massage the back.

22. How would you instruct a client to use the hydrotherapy facilities of the spa or health club during his or her visit there for a massage session? Include timing relative to the massage, amount of time to stay in them, and other safety precautions. Limit to two different types of facilities.

Sample Answer: I would instruct the client that the hydrotherapy facilities are best used before the massage. That would begin the relaxation process. For thermo-therapies like steam room and whirlpool, I would recommend that they shower before using the facilities and limit their use to 10–30 minutes (depending on their age and general health). I would also suggest that they not eat for at least 30 minutes before using the facilities and that they should drink plenty of liquids before, during, and afterward.

Before I gave them a massage, I would be sure that they felt well, were cooled down, and had been drinking water.

CHAPTER 12 MYOFASCIAL MASSAGE

1. c

2. b

3. a

4. c

5. b

6. c

7. b

8. b

9. c

10. a

11. Name and describe the three different types of fascia distinguished as being at different depths in the body.

   Sample Answer: Fascia at different depths in the body are (1) *superficial fascia,* which is a continuous layer of connective tissue over the entire body between the skin and deep fascia; (2) *deep fascia,* which is an intricate series of dense connective tissue sheets and bands that hold muscles, organs, and other structures in place throughout the body; and (3) *subserous fascia,* which lies between deep fascia and the serous membranes lining the body cavities.

12. Identify and explain four functions of fascia in the body.

   Sample Answer: Four functions of fascia in the body are (1) holds structures together and gives them their characteristic shapes, (2) separates tissues (e.g., individual muscles), (3) plays a part in cellular respiration, and (4) connects the body as a whole in a continuous sheet of fascia.

13. Explain the metaphor of fascia as a knitted sweater.

   Sample Answer: Fascia is sometimes compared to a knitted sweater. In a sweater all of the threads of yarn are connected in interwoven patterns, and a pull in one section of a sweater causes a pull in the entire sweater affecting spots distant from the original pull. This distorts the entire sweater. Fascia is like this in connecting the entire body with winding sheets, and a distortion or adhesion in one place causes distortion throughout and at distant points in the body.

14. Explain how myofascial techniques release adhesions and result in more pliable tissues.

   Sample Answer: Myofascial techniques warm and stretch fascial tissues so that they are more pliable. This is the principle of thixotropy at work. The slow horizontal stretching of tissues breaks cross-links between fascial sheets, unsticking the tissues and increasing local circulation.

15. Describe four important guidelines for performing myofascial massage.

Sample Answer: I think that the four most important guidelines for performing myofascial massage are (1) using gentle contact and entering the tissues slowly, (2) moving the tissues horizontally, (3) maintaining a continuous stretch, (4) waiting for a feeling of "melting" or subtle movement in the tissues.

CHAPTER 13 NEUROMUSCULAR THERAPY (NMT): TRIGGER POINTS

1. b
2. d
3. a
4. b
5. c
6. a
7. c
8. b
9. a
10. c

11. Give six examples of autonomic phenomena that can be "triggered" by active trigger points.

Sample Answer: Six examples of autonomic phenomena that can be triggered by active trigger points are (1) pain, (2) spasm, (3) vasoconstriction, (4) goose bumps, (5) vasodilation, and (6) sweating.

12. Discuss how trigger points are activated. Include both direct and indirect stimuli.

Sample Answer: Trigger points can be activated by a number of stimuli (e.g., directly by overwork of a muscle, chilling, or gross trauma; indirectly by arthritis, emotional distress, or certain diseases).

13. Describe methods of locating trigger points on a client/patient.

Sample Answer: Trigger points may be located on a client/patient by palpation of a tender spot with taut band, information from a client about recent muscle overload or trauma, inference from observation of a client's posture, or client marking x on a chart where he or she feels pain.

14. Describe in detail the method of deactivating a trigger point using ischemic compression. Include point location, application of pressure, knowing when the point has released, and finishing.

Sample Answer: Deactivating a trigger point involves four steps: (1) locating the TrP by palpation of a tender spot and taut band or by information provided by the recipient, (2) using the thumb or hand tool to apply pressure to the exact spot (i.e., on the taut band) with enough pressure to cause blanching with hypoxia and holding for 20–60 seconds until the TrP releases, (3) feeling for release of the TrP, which will be palpated as a softening of the spot and as a decrease in sensation and pain as reported by the recipient; (4) finishing deactivation with a stretch of the affected muscle to return it to its normal length.

15. Identify at least three different manual methods of deactivating a trigger point besides ischemic compression.

Sample Answer: Trigger points can be deactivated using manual methods other than ischemic compression, including deep stroking or stripping over the area, deep friction at the TrP site, pinching the TrP between the finger and the thumb in muscles structured appropriately, and vibration over the TrP.

CHAPTER 14 LYMPHATIC DRAINAGE MASSAGE

1. b
2. b
3. d
4. d
5. c
6. c
7. b
8. a
9. c
10. c

11. Draw a diagram of the initial lymphatics (i.e., lymph capillaries) and label important parts of the structure. Explain how lymphatic drainage massage techniques facilitate the flow of lymph fluid into these tiny vessels.

Sample Answer: (See Figure 14-1 for diagram of initial lymphatics.) Lymphatic drainage massage techniques move the superficial skin layers, which pulls on the anchoring filaments attached to the cell walls, which opens the overflaps between cells, which allows lymph fluid to enter the tiny vessels.

12. Draw an outline of a person and indicate (and label) major lymph node locations. Using arrows to indicate direction, draw the pattern of lymph movement toward the thoracic and right lymphatic ducts (label location of ducts).

Sample Answer: (See Figure 14-2 for schematic drawing of the lymph system.)

13. Explain the importance of pressure, direction, rhythm, and sequence when applying lymphatic drainage techniques.

Sample Answer: In applying lymphatic drainage massage techniques, it is important to use light *pressure* (i.e., only enough to create traction to move the skin). Too much pressure closes off the overflaps of the initial lymphatics and prevents lymph fluid from entering them. The movement is performed in the *direction* of the targeted lymph node. The *rhythm* of application includes an active phase in which skin is moved in the desired direction, and then a passive phase when the skin snaps back to its original position. This is repeated with an even rhythm 6–8 times in each spot. Finally, the *sequence* is determined by the body's lymph drainage pathways so that fluid moves in the direction of the left and right thoracic ducts and is returned to the cardiovascular system.

14. Describe in detail one of the lymphatic drainage massage techniques.

Sample Answer: In the *stationary circles* technique, the fingertips pads are placed lightly on the skin with just enough pressure to create traction and move superficial skin layers. Hands are places side-by-side so that the eight fingers are lined up and are flat against the skin. Fingertips make a circular movement, with the first or active phase in the shape of an L toward the targeted lymph node, and the remainder of the circle a passive phase or "riding" the skin back to the beginning spot. The fingers do not slide over the skin but move the skin in a circular pattern.

CHAPTER 15 FOOT REFLEXOLOGY

1. c
2. b
3. d
4. a
5. c
6. d
7. a
8. d
9. b
10. c
11. Explain how the theory of Zone Therapy relates to the reflexology maps of the feet.

Sample Answer 1: While Zone Therapy provides the theoretical framework when looking at the body as a whole, reflexology maps are practical guides to what structures lay in specific zones and where to apply pressure to the feet.

Sample Answer 2: Reflexology maps indicate which body structures are affected by pressure on specific spots on the feet. Those body structures can be found in the longitudinal zone that ends in that spot on the feet according to Zone Therapy theory.

12. Draw outlines of right and left foot bottoms. Be sure to draw the toes clearly to distinguish between the two feet. Draw in and label the following body structures in their correct locations on the feet according to the theory of reflexology: lung, sinuses, shoulders, heart, liver, stomach, kidney, and large intestine.

Sample Answer: (See Figure 15-1 for foot reflexology chart.)

CHAPTER 16 POLARITY THERAPY

1. c
2. b
3. a
4. b
5. c
6. b

7. c

8. c

9. a

10. d

11. Describe some of the objective changes that have been observed in recipients of Polarity Therapy that indicate that the session is having a physiological effect.

> Sample Answer: Objective physiological effects that have been observed in recipients of Polarity Therapy include signs of deep relaxation (e.g., cheeks flush, blood pressure drops, salivation increases, heart rate slows, eyes tear, stomach grumbles). Gentle rocking motions stimulate mechanoreceptors in the joints resulting in lower muscle tone, increased local circulation, freer joint movement, reduced pain, and release of endorphins for feeling of well-being.

12. Discuss the concept of *energy* in the context of Polarity Therapy. Describe what a Polarity Therapy practitioner feels as an indication of energy movement or obstruction.

> Sample Answer: The concept of *energy* in Polarity Therapy may be described in esoteric terms using the writings of Randolph Stone, which are based partly on ancient Indian (i.e., Ayurvedic) medicine. In this framework *energy* is the life force or "prana" that moves in the body in energy centers called charkas. *Energy* may also be thought of in more general terms as a life force that flows in the body and must remain free flowing for good health. This *energy* is felt by the practitioner as tingling in the hands or as a presence or sensation when the hands are held or moved slightly above the body. Obstructions in energy flow are felt as stagnation or holding or tension.

CHAPTER 17 ASIAN BODYWORK THERAPY- THEORY

1. d

2. b

3. c

4. c

5. Yang

6. Yang

7. Yin

8. Yin

9. a

10. a

11. c

12. d

13. b

14. c

15. b

16. c

17. a

18. c

19. c

20. b

21. Contrast traditional Chinese medicine with Western scientific medicine. How does each view the body? An individuals place in the universe? The nature of health and disease?

Sample Answer: Traditional Chinese medicine evolved over centuries from experience and observation; developed a theory of energy (Qi) flow and system of energy channels and acupoints; views humans as an integral part of a dynamic universe that is ever changing yet maintaining unity; and focuses on restoring energy (Qi) balance for maintaining health and preventing disease. Its major methods are herbs, acupuncture, exercises (qi gong, tai chi), and Asian bodywork therapies such as tuina and acupressure. Western medicine is based primarily on scientific experimentation and knowledge of Western anatomy, physiology, and pathology; views humans in a more mechanistic way with separation of body and mind; and excels in emergency breakdown repairs to the body. Western medicine views disease in terms of breakdown of function in the systems of the body (e.g., digestive or respiratory) and of invasion of the body by viruses and bacteria. Its major methods include drugs and surgery, although more focus is currently being placed on lifestyle changes such as diet and exercise.

22. Draw the Yin/Yang symbol, and explain its meaning. Identify the nature of Yin and Yang and the five principles of interaction between them.

Sample Answer: (See Figure 17-3 for Yin/Yang symbol.) The *Yin/Yang symbol* depicts the relatedness and interconnectedness of all and the constant movement and change in the universe. It symbolizes the dynamic relationship between Yin (dark side) and Yang (light side) as they influence and flow into each other. A dot of Yin on the Yang side and a dot of Yang on the Yin side show that these principles are not a strict dichotomy but that a little bit of each is also present in the opposite. *Yin* is dark, deep, dense, feminine, interior, still, substantial, cool and contracting compared to Yang. *Yang* is light, energetic, ethereal, masculine, exterior, moving warm and expanding compared to Yin. The five principles of interaction between Yin and Yang are opposition, interdependence, consuming/supporting relationship, intertransformation, and infinite divisibility.

23. Name and describe the five functions of Qi.

Sample Answer: The five functions of Qi are (1) *transforms* nutrients so that the body can use them (e.g., digesting food), (2) *transports* nutrients throughout the body and regulates the flow of emotions, (3) *holds* everything together and helps body maintain integrity, (4) *protects* the body by energizing the immune system, (5) *warms* the body and regulates metabolism.

24. Explain the proper use of acupoints in Asian bodywork therapy.

Sample Answer: Acupoints are used for diagnosis and treatment of energy imbalances. They are points at which energy channels can be best accessed for application of acupuncture and acupressure techniques. Acupoints are used in balancing energy (e.g., removing obstructions or dispersing excess) as a preventative health measure. A less effective use of acupoints is for treatment of specific symptoms in the Western medical model.

CHAPTER 18 AMMA—TRADITIONAL JAPANESE MASSAGE

1. c

2. b

3. a

4. d
5. c
6. c
7. b
8. d
9. a
10. c

CHAPTER 19 ZEN SHIATSU: AN OVERVIEW

1. b
2. d
3. a
4. d
5. b
6. e
7. a
8. c
9. c
10. a
11. b
12. b
13. b
14. c
15. c
16. b
17. d
18. c

CHAPTER 20 JIN SHIN DO®

1. c
2. b
3. d
4. b
5. c
6. a
7. d
8. b
9. b
10. a

CHAPTER 21 SPORTS AND FITNESS

1. c

2. e

3. a

4. d

5. c

6. b

7. c

8. c

9. a

10. d

11. Distinguish among maintenance, remedial, and rehabilitation sports massage using examples for clarification.

   Sample Answer: *Maintenance* sports massage is received regularly by an athlete to help them keep in top performance and prevent injuries, and it focuses on recovery and remedial treatment. An example is a runner who receives massage regularly as part of his or her training plan. *Remedial* sports massage address problem conditions that, if allowed to progress, would result in injuries (e.g., deactivating trigger points that are shortening and weakening muscles). *Rehabilitation* sports massage is used to help an athlete heal from a disabling injury (e.g., lymphatic drainage massage to help reduce swelling around a sprained ankle).

12. Name forms of hydrotherapy typically available in gyms and health clubs. Describe how different forms of hydrotherapy can be used to enhance the effects of recovery massage.

   Sample Answer: Forms of hydrotherapy typically available in gyms and health clubs include hot showers, whirlpool, steam room, and sauna. These enhance the effects of recovery massage by promoting general and muscular relaxation, by increasing elimination of metabolic wastes through sweating, and by increasing general circulation. They are best used before a massage session.

13. Describe in detail the application of pre-event sports massage including goals of the session, duration, types of massage techniques used, and other important factors.

   Sample Answer: The goals of a pre-event sports massage are to prepare the athlete physically and mentally for competition. Specific goals include warming muscle tissues, freeing joints, increasing circulation, and stimulating mental clarity. The pre-event session is about 15 minutes in duration, fast paced, upbeat, and stimulating. Techniques used for pre-event massage include rhythmic compression, kneading, direct pressure to stress points, jostling, and joint movements. Focus is on muscles most important for the upcoming event.

14. Describe in detail the application of postevent sports massage including goals of the session, duration, types of massage techniques used, and other important factors.

   Sample Answer: The goals of a postevent sports massage session are to help the athlete recover physically and psychologically from a specific sports event and identify possible injuries suffered in the competition. Specific goals include muscular relaxation, flushing tissues of metabolic wastes, and returning to a state of relaxation and calm. A postevent massage session immediately after an event is about 15 minutes in length, slower paced, gentler, and calmer. Techniques used for postevent massage include rhythmic compressions, kneading, direct pressure, and joint movements. Focus is on muscles stressed in the event.

15. Choose a specific sport or fitness activity (e.g., running, swimming, tennis, baseball, golf, bowling, soccer, bicycling) for this exercise. Describe how the nature of the sport would affect your plan for maintenance massage of an athlete who participates in the activity regularly.

   Sample Answer: The athlete is a *golfer*. Since golf is a warm weather sport, the athlete would be most active as a golfer in the spring and summer (in a temperate climate with four distinct seasons) with one or two trips to warmer climates in the winter to golf. During the golf season, and after a golf trip in the winter, a maintenance session would include specific attention to the arm and shoulder muscles looking for stresses and strains, particularly around tendons in the elbow. Deep transverse friction on affected tendons and stretching of shoulder and arms would be included. Special attention to the lower back would also be appropriate for a golfer. During the off-season, maintenance sports massage would focus on recovery from old injuries and improving tissue pliability and flexibility (i.e., recovery from the past season and preparing for the upcoming season).

CHAPTER 22 MOTHER AND CHILD

1. c
2. b
3. d
4. b
5. a
6. b
7. b
8. c
9. a
10. c
11. a
12. c
13. b
14. d
15. c

16. Describe the typical pregnancy posture, and identify the stresses it creates on the body. Explain how this affects the goals for pregnancy massage.

   Sample Answer: Typical pregnancy posture can be described as head forward, chest back, belly out, hips tilted forward, locked knees, and feet turned out. This creates undue stress particularly in the neck and lower back. One of the goals of pregnancy massage is to relieve stress and relax muscles in the neck and lower back.

17. List at least five potential benefits of pregnancy massage.

   Sample Answer: Five potential benefits of pregnancy massage are (1) releasing emotional stress, (2) relieving physical stress in neck and lower back, (3) reducing swelling in the limbs, (4) reducing overall muscle soreness, (5) reducing postnatal complications.

18. Describe how you would set up an ideal environment for pregnancy massage. List at least five factors that you would take into consideration.

> Sample Answer: Five factors important for an ideal environment for pregnancy massage are (1) cooler room temperature, (2) fresh flowing air, (3) toilet nearby, (4) plenty of bolsters for comfortable positioning, (5) relaxing atmosphere.

19. Identify at least five contraindications or cautions for pregnancy massage.

> Sample Answer: Five contraindications for pregnancy massage are (1) high-risk pregnancy, (2) morning sickness or any nausea, (3) vomiting, (4) vaginal bleeding, (5) pain in the abdomen.

20. Describe the four major possibilities for positioning a pregnant recipient for massage. Discuss when you would use each one, and when you would avoid it.

> Sample Answer: Four primary position choices for pregnancy massage include (1) *prone* during first few months of pregnancy, (2) *supine* during first few months of pregnancy, but avoided once fetus grows, (3) *reclining* at any time but good alternative to supine after first few months, (4) *side-lying* at any time. (A fifth choice might be *seated* if lying down or getting on the table is too difficult for some reason.)

CHAPTER 23 HEALTHY AGING

1. c
2. a
3. d
4. c
5. a
6. b
7. b
8. d
9. c
10. c

11. List eight common physical effects of aging.

> Sample Answer: Eight common physical effects of aging are (1) decrease in mobility and strength, (2) slower nerve conduction, (3) less connective tissue elasticity, (4) thinner and dryer skin, (5) loss of bone mass, (6) poorer eyesight, (7) poorer hearing, (8) less effective immune system.

12. Explain the special benefits of massage for the elderly population.

> Sample Answer: Massage has special benefits for elderly people. In addition to keeping tissues healthy and anatomical systems functioning well, massage can help elders with maintaining the flexibility and strength needed for daily living activities such as walking, getting into and out of the bathtub, and standing up from sitting in a chair. Massage can address some of the special problems of aging, such as dry skin and poor bowel movement. Massage also provides a social outlet for isolated elderly and a caring touch needed by people at any age. Loss, frustration, fear, and grief experienced especially by institutionalized elderly can be alleviated with the anxiety and stress reduction resulting from massage.

13. Summarize the findings of research on the benefits of massage for the institutionalized elderly.

Sample Answer: Research on the benefits of massage for the institutionalized elderly showed that massage provides relaxation and improved communication and reduces the dehumanizing effects of institutionalization. Back massage seemed particularly useful.

14. Name the three physiological age categories for the elderly, and describe characteristics of people in each category. Explain massage considerations for each category.

Sample Answer: The three physiological categories for the elderly are (1) *Robust* elderly, who exhibit few of the normal signs of aging. Robust elders can be approached as most middle-aged massage recipients. (2) *Age appropriate* elders, who exhibit many of the typical effects of aging. A thorough health history is needed to identify contraindications, and massage application should be gentler to avoid damaging tissues. (3) *Frail* elderly, who look and feel fragile. Frail elders need special care and much gentler massage application, including lighter pressure and slower joint movement and help getting onto and off of the massage table.

15. List at least five goals for massage for healthy aging, and describe the techniques appropriate for achieving each goal.

Sample Answer: Five goals for healthy aging are (1) improved fluid circulation through effleurage, kneading, and jostling techniques, (2) more pliable connective tissues through kneading, compression, joint mobilizing, and stretching techniques, (3) greater flexibility through muscle relaxation and stretching techniques, (4) better elimination through abdominal massage, (5) more upright posture aided by lengthening (relaxing and stretching) the muscles on the front of the body especially the abdominal and pectoral muscles.

CHAPTER 24 TERMINALLY ILL AND DYING

1. c
2. b
3. b
4. d
5. c
6. a
7. b
8. a
9. c
10. b

11. List the most important physical, emotional, and social benefits of massage for the terminally ill and dying.

Sample Answer: The most important physical benefits for massage for the terminally ill and dying include general relaxation, improved fluid circulation, muscle relaxation, and skin health especially for those bed-ridden for a long time. Common problems such as insomnia, constipation, difficulty breathing, and skin degeneration can be alleviated by massage. Emotional and social benefits include social contact, anxiety reduction, lessening isolation and depression, release of emotional tension, and increased feeling of well-being.

12. Explain how in the wellness model, someone who is terminally ill can be said to be striving for high-level wellness despite that fact that he or she is going to die soon.

Sample Answer: From a wellness perspective, we are constantly striving for optimal well-being in many dimensions of our lives (e.g., physical, mental, emotional, social, and spiritual). Wellness focuses on the *quality* of life, not necessarily longevity. So while the physical body may be close to death, a person can still experience well-being in other aspects of his or her life.

13. Describe the qualities and techniques of massage for sessions with the terminally ill and dying.

Sample Answer: Massage sessions with the terminally ill and dying are shorter, softer, and gentler. Techniques vary from simple hand holding to full-body massage depending on the condition of the recipient. Recipients may be seated, in hospital or regular beds, or on massage tables. There may be more verbal communication if recipients need to talk, or sessions may be silent, facilitating nonverbal communication. Sessions are specially tailored for the needs of each unique recipient.

14. List the benefits of hand and arm massage for the terminally ill and dying. Describe the qualities and techniques of the massage.

Sample Answer: Hand and arm massage is a good approach when getting to know a new recipient and for nonprofessional caregivers to perform. People are used to having their hands and arms touched, so it is a safe introduction to massage, and there are fewer contraindications and endangerment sites associated with the arms and hands. Holding the hands is comforting to most people and affords the opportunity for eye contact. Techniques are gentle and include applying lotion with effleurage, kneading the forearms, joint movements in the wrist and hands, gently squeezing the fingers, and effleurage (long strokes) from hand to elbow.

15. Describe a holistic self-care strategy when working with the terminally ill and dying.

Sample Answer: A self-care strategy when working with the terminally ill and dying has both physical and emotional aspects. Physical self-care involves special attention to body mechanics when working in unusual circumstances (e.g., by a hospital bed) and in protecting yourself from communicable disease. Emotional self-care involves working through feelings about death and dying and your clients with a coworker, friend, or supervisor.

CHAPTER 25 SEATED MASSAGE IN THE WORKPLACE

1. d
2. c
3. b
4. b
5. d
6. b
7. Explain the popularity of workplace massage. Identify at least four important factors.

Sample Answer: Workplace massage is popular for a number of different reasons, including (1) it has immediate positive results as recipients feel better right away, (2) it alleviates some of the aches and pains from sitting for long periods of time at desks, (3) it does not require practice or effort, (4) it complements other health practices, such as weight reduction and exercise programs.

8. Summarize the benefits of massage both to the individual worker and to the employer.

Sample Answer: The benefits of massage to the individual worker include overall stress reduction, improved circulation, muscle relaxation (especially in the upper body), specific attention to areas of repetitive strain, and increase in mental alertness and feelings of well-being. Benefits to the employer include improved worker productivity, increased loyalty and positive feelings toward the workplace, healthier workers, and reduced absenteeism.

9. Give an example of a worker who could benefit from workplace massage. Describe his or her job, work station, and specific benefits of massage for his or her situation.

Sample Answer: An example of a worker who could benefit from workplace massage is a computer programmer. His or her job involves sitting for long periods of time, upper-body muscular strain, and mental fatigue. The work station is a desk with computer and keyboard, and manuals and other reference material. Special benefits of massage for a computer programmer are general stress reduction; improved circulation; reduction of muscle tension and trigger points in the shoulders, arms, and hands; reduction of tension in the neck (e.g., tension headache); increased mental clarity and rejuvenation.

10. Describe a seated massage session for the workplace. Include the duration, the goals, the techniques used, and the general sequence of the routine.

Sample Answer: Seated massage for the workplace is typically 15–20 minutes in duration. Goals include general relaxation, muscular relaxation in upper body, improved circulation, increased mental clarity, and feelings of revitalization. Massage techniques chosen are those appropriate for use over clothing (e.g., compression, pressure points kneading, vibration, friction, joint movements, and tapotement or percussion). A general sequence for a seated massage routine might be to begin with massage of back and shoulders, then arms and hands, neck and head, and finish with tapotement overall for stimulation and preparing to go back to work.

Video Segment Questions

1. BODY MECHANICS

1. To determine proper table height, stand at the side of the table with hands hanging down. The table should be at your
   a. elbows
   b. fingertips
   c. first or second knuckles
   d. wrists

2. Lower your body by bending at the
   a. waist
   b. knees
   c. neck
   d. shoulders

3. Apply pressure by
   a. shifting the weight
   b. pushing with the arms
   c. bending at the waist
   d. extending the wrist

4. The wrist should be kept in this position as much as possible to avoid strain.
   a. flexion
   b. hyperextension
   c. neutral
   d. abducted

5. To avoid strain when applying thumb pressure, be sure that thumb and wrist joints are
   a. at right angles
   b. hyperextended
   c. flexed
   d. in straight alignment

6. During compression techniques, the reinforcing hand is placed over the bottom hand's
   a. fingers
   b. metacarpals

c. wrist

d. lower arm

7. Briefly describe proper body mechanics while sitting.

8. Describe two stances to use while performing massage.

2. POSITIONING AND DRAPING

1. When the recipient is supine, place bolsters
   a. under the knees and shoulders
   b. under the knees and neck
   c. under the ankles and hips
   d. under the ankles and wrists

2. When the recipient is prone, place bolsters
   a. under the knees and shoulders
   b. under the knees and neck
   c. under the ankles and shoulders
   d. under the hips and shoulders

3. When a recipient is in side-lying position, place bolsters
   a. under the head, bent upper leg, and upper arm
   b. under the head, straight lower leg, and upper elbow
   c. under the lower ankle, upper hip, and upper arm
   d. under the head, lower knee, and lower hip

4. The genitals and women's breasts are
   a. draped when the room is cold
   b. draped unless they prefer to be undraped
   c. draped at all times
   d. undraped when requested

5. The technique used to secure the drape when the recipient is turning over is called
   a. tucking
   b. tenting
   c. shifting
   d. pinning

6. Explain the purposes of good draping.

7. List the guidelines for good draping.

3. INTRODUCTION TO WESTERN MASSAGE

1. Match the following Western massage techniques with the descriptions below.

   a. effleurage
   b. petrissage
   c. friction
   d. tapotement
   e. vibration
   f. touch without movement
      kneading
      trembling

holding
sliding
percussion
rubbing together

4. EFFLEURAGE

1. Effleurage techniques are strokes that
   a. lift and wring
   b. oscillate
   c. rub together
   d. slide and glide

2. The pressure used for effleurage techniques should
   a. always be light
   b. begin light and gradually deepen
   c. begin deep and fast
   d. never vary

3. The amount of oil used for effleurage should be
   a. plentiful for maximum slide
   b. slippery for smooth strokes
   c. limited to what is necessary
   d. generous for least traction

4. For body areas with dry skin or a lot of hair, the amount of oil used should be
   a. increased to avoid pulling
   b. decreased to avoid chaffing
   c. minimal for best effect
   d. less than usual

5. Deep effleurage is best applied to broad areas like the back using the
   a. fingertips
   b. palms
   c. knuckles
   d. forearm

6. List the uses of effleurage techniques during massage.

7. Describe the general effects of effleurage techniques.

5. PETRISSAGE

1. Petrissage techniques
   a. slide and glide
   b. rub and warm
   c. lift or compress
   d. oscillate or tremble

2. The oil or lotion used for petrissage techniques should be
   a. generous and thick
   b. slippery and smooth

    c. thick and moisturizing
    d. minimal and light

3. Bruising and pinching may result from using
    a. too much pressure
    b. too much oil
    c. not enough pressure
    d. correct pressure

4. When performing compression with the palms of the hands, avoid
    a. full contact with the palms
    b. rhythmic movement
    c. hyper-extending the wrists
    d. reinforcing with one hand over the other

5. Skin rolling involves
    a. compressing skin tissues
    b. lifting the skin from tissues underneath
    c. sliding over the skin
    d. vibrating the skin

6. Describe effects of petrissage techniques.

7. List important principles of applying petrissage techniques.

6. FRICTION

1. Superficial friction causes
    a. better lymph flow
    b. warming of skin tissues
    c. separation of fibers
    d. better scar formation

2. To prevent chaffing during superficial friction, be careful of
    a. the direction of movement
    b. the rhythm of movement
    c. the amount of pressure used
    d. the part of the hand used

3. During deep friction techniques, the fingers should not
    a. slide over the skin
    b. move the skin over deeper tissues
    c. create friction between tissue layers
    d. contact the skin firmly

4. In applying Cyriax friction to a sheathed tendon, the tendon should be
    a. soft and relaxed
    b. shortened and relaxed
    c. on maximum stretch
    d. on minimum stretch

5. Before and/or after Cyriax friction, use this modality on the site.
    a. ice
    b. hot pack
    c. electrical stimulation
    d. electrical vibration

6. Describe three directions for applying deep friction techniques.

7. Explain the desired effects for deep transverse or Cyriax friction.

7. TAPOTEMENT

1. Tapotement techniques are also known as
   a. sliding
   b. percussion
   c. vibration
   d. stroking

2. The proper application of tapotement is best described as
   a. heavy, slow, penetrating
   b. vigorous, jarring, painful
   c. rapid, heavy, penetrating
   d. light, rapid, rhythmic

3. Variations of tapotement are created by
   a. using different parts of the hands
   b. slowing the pace
   c. changing the rhythm
   d. changing the force of application

4. A variation of tapotement used to treat lung congestion is
   a. tapping
   b. quacking
   c. cupping
   d. rapping

5. A variation of tapotement appropriate for use on the head is
   a. tapping
   b. rapping
   c. cupping
   d. hacking

6. Describe the use of tapotement techniques during massage.

7. Explain the effects of tapotement techniques.

8. VIBRATION

1. Fine vibration is performed manually
   a. over a large area with the palm
   b. across joints with the whole hand
   c. over a small area with the fingertips
   d. over a broad area with the forearm

2. Fine vibration is generated by the practitioner using tension in the
   a. forearms
   b. shoulders
   c. hands
   d. back

3. Fine vibration over the abdomen is used
   a. to improve breathing

b. to stimulate digestion and elimination

c. for general relaxation

d. to improve mental clarity

4. A type of coarse vibration involving joint movement as muscles of a limb are tossed from hand to hand is

a. stretching

b. shaking

c. jostling

d. bilateral tree stroking

5. A form of coarse vibration used to relieve tension in an individual muscle is

a. shaking

b. stretching

c. quacking

d. rolling

6. Describe desirable features of a professional electronic massager.

7. Explain the physiological effects of fine and coarse vibration.

9. TOUCH WITHOUT MOVEMENT

1. Touch without movement may be described as

a. casual touch with no special intention

b. social touch with no special intention

c. skilled touch with specific therapeutic intention

d. casual touch with social intention

2. Passive touch and holding are used during massage for

a. stimulation and transition

b. calming and integration

c. increasing circulation and tissue pliability

d. muscle relaxation and lymphatic flow

3. An example of touch without movement used as a finishing technique on a supine recipient is

a. passive touch on the back

b. jostling the leg

c. holding the feet

d. tapping the head

4. List several possible purposes for the use of touch without movement during massage.

5. Identify places on the body where passive touch and holding are commonly applied at the end of a massage session as finishing techniques.

10. JOINT MOVEMENTS

1. Mobilizing techniques involve the free movement of joints

a. beyond their normal range of motion

b. to the limit of their range of motion

c. well within their normal range

d. outside of their normal range

2. Mobilizing techniques can be described as

a. free, loose, smooth

b. controlled, precise, rhythmic
c. loose, precise, elongating
d. smooth, controlled, elongating

3. Stretching techniques involve
   a. taking a joint beyond the limit of its range of motion
   b. elongating soft tissues around a joint
   c. shaking a limb to relax surrounding muscles
   d. free and relaxed movements

4. Before stretching, perform the following for best results:
   a. apply ice to the tissues to be stretched
   b. crack the joint to free it up
   c. warm surrounding soft tissues
   d. force the joint beyond its normal range

5. The following movements are *not* within the scope of massage therapy:
   a. mobilizing techniques within the normal range
   b. stretching techniques to the limit of normal range
   c. stretching techniques to elongate soft tissues surrounding joints
   c. forced joint movements beyond normal range

6. List several potential effects of joint movements.

7. Discuss safety precautions for performing joint movements.

11. MYOFASCIAL MASSAGE

1. The goal of myofascial massage is to
   a. improve general circulation
   b. calm nerves surrounding fascial tissues
   c. separate adhering fascial tissues
   d. improve joint function

2. An important principle of performance in myofascial massage is to
   a. make forceful contact
   b. enter the tissues slowly
   c. use deep pressure
   d. pull tissues apart quickly

3. Once the desired depth of penetration is reached, tissues are stretched
   a. vertically
   b. perpendicularly
   c. diagonally
   d. horizontally

4. Tissues are stretched slowly until you feel
   a. a taut band
   b. a point of resistance
   c. ropey tissues
   d. a pulse

5. Hold the stretch of tissues until you feel
   a. resistance to the stretch
   b. a giving or elongation of tissues
   c. a contraction of tissues
   d. a sudden snap

6. Describe the goals of myofascial massage.

7. List some of the health problems caused by adhering myofascial tissues.

12. NEUROMUSCULAR THERAPY

1. To the practitioner, trigger points feel like
   a. soft spots in muscles
   b. taut bands of tissue
   c. depressions in tendons
   d. soft spots in tendons

2. When pressed, active trigger points refer pain to their
   a. trigger zone
   b. active zone
   c. latent zone
   d. reference zone

3. Trigger points are deactivated using a manual technique called
   a. ischemic compression
   b. rhythmic compression
   c. point palpation
   d. point stretch

4. Trigger points are located by palpation *and*
   a. visual inspection of skin
   b. feeling for restrictions
   c. feed back from recipient
   d. electrical impulse

5. When a trigger point deactivates, the practitioner will feel
   a. hardening of tissues
   b. softening of tissues
   c. stringy bands
   d. circular bands

6. List negative effects of active trigger points.

7. Identify common causes of trigger points.

13. LYMPHATIC DRAINAGE MASSAGE

1. Lymphatic massage techniques are
   a. firm, fast, forceful
   b. slow, light, repetitive
   c. fast, light, precise
   d. heavy, slow, penetrating

2. Lymphatic massage techniques cause the flow of intercellular fluid into
   a. arteries
   b. veins
   c. larger lymph vessels
   d. lymph capillaries

3. The pressure used when performing lymphatic massage should be
    a. just enough to move the skin
    b. enough to increase blood circulation
    c. enough to move muscle tissue
    d. enough to move lymph in larger vessels

4. In lymphatic massage, the direction of movement for each technique is toward
    a. the heart
    b. the thoracic duct
    c. the targeted lymph node
    d. the aorta

5. This performance error will close off the lymph capillaries
    a. using repetitive movements
    b. using too light pressure
    c. using too heavy pressure
    d. allowing the skin to snap back

6. Explain how lymphatic massage improves the function of the lymphatic system.

14. REFLEXOLOGY

1. Pressure on specific spots on the feet is thought to stimulate
    a. deep relaxation
    b. greater mental clarity
    c. improved sense of well-being
    d. corresponding areas in other parts of the body

2. Reflexology techniques and charts were developed in the 1940s by
    a. Pehr Ling
    b. Eunice Ingham
    c. Randolph Stone
    d. Mary McMillan

3. This technique is used to press points systematically and quickly.
    a. hook and backup
    b. direct pressure
    c. thumb walking
    d. squeezing

4. This technique is used for deep pressure to a specific spot.
    a. hook and backup
    b. thumb walking
    c. finger waking
    d. joint movement

5. List some physiological effects of reflexology.

15. POLARITY THERAPY

1. The goal of polarity therapy is to
    a. remove restrictions in myofascial tissues
    b. improve the flow of lymph

    c. remove obstructions to energy flow

    d. polarize the body and limbs

2. Many of the beneficial physiological effects of polarity therapy can be traced to

    a. improved blood circulation

    b. mind and body relaxation

    c. electrical stimulation

    d. kinesthetic awareness

3. Polarity therapy can be described as

    a. simple touch and gentle movements

    b. simple touch and vigorous movements

    c. slow repetitive movements

    d. fast-paced rhythmic movements

4. Major polarity therapy techniques are

    a. rocking, direct pressure, touch without movement

    b. effleurage, petrissage, tapotement

    c. scoop, pump, stationary circles

    d. friction, holding, stretching

5. Each polarity therapy technique is held or performed for

    a. 10–15 seconds

    b. 20–30 seconds

    c. 1–2 minutes

    d. 5–7 minutes

16. ACUPRESSURE TECHNIQUE

1. The intent of Asian bodywork is to

    a. improve blood circulation

    b. facilitate the flow of chi

    c. realign posture

    d. elicit general relaxation

2. The four pillars of assessment in Asian bodywork are

    a. pressing, shaking, asking, telling

    b. stroking, pressing, percussion, moxibustion

    c. ying, yang, wood, chi

    d. seeing, touching, hearing/smelling, asking

3. For good body mechanics when performing Asian bodywork on a massage table, set the table height

    a. the same as Western massage

    b. lower than Western massage

    c. higher than Western massage

    d. on the last setting

4. In Asian bodywork, pressure is applied to acupoints using

    a. weight transfer

    b. arm strength

    c. shoulder strength

    d. leg strength

5. The correct angle of penetration of acupoints is
   a. 30 degrees
   b. 45 degrees
   c. 90 degrees
   d. 120 degrees

6. List four principles of good body mechanics for applying pressure to acupoints.

17. SPORTS MASSAGE

1. The primary goal of pre-event sports massage is
   a. recovery
   b. rehabilitation
   c. readiness
   d. relaxation

2. Pre-event massage can be described as
   a. upbeat, short, fast paced
   b. soothing, short, slow paced
   c. comforting, relaxing, moderately paced
   d. oily, smooth, relaxing

3. The primary goal of postevent massage is
   a. readiness
   b. rehabilitation
   c. recovery
   d. flexibility

4. This technique would not be used in postevent massage
   a. kneading
   b. compression
   c. jostling
   d. percussion

5. The pressure used in postevent massage is
   a. the same as pre-event massage
   b. heavier than pre-event massage
   c. lighter than pre-event massage
   d. as light as you can make it

6. List massage techniques used in pre-event massage.

7. Describe what to look for in determining whether an athlete is ready for postevent massage.

18. PREGNANCY MASSAGE

1. Pregnancy massage is
   a. vigorous and stimulating
   b. gentle and relaxing
   c. relaxing but painful
   d. gentle but stimulating

2. Typical pregnancy posture causes strain in the
   a. toes
   b. upper back

    c. lower back
    d. ankles

3. The arms and legs of pregnant women are commonly
    a. swollen
    b. cold
    c. relaxed
    d. spongy

4. Avoid massage of this area in pregnant women
    a. feet
    b. abdomen
    c. shoulders
    d. hands

5. List the benefits of massage for pregnant women.

6. Describe the placement of bolsters for pregnant women in the side-lying position.

7. Identify contraindications for pregnancy massage.

19. INFANT MASSAGE

1. Massage helps the development of a baby's nervous system through
    a. the oil applied
    b. relief of trigger points
    c. tactile stimulation and movement
    d. improving digestion and elimination

2. The oil used for infant massage should be
    a. unscented
    b. lavender scented
    c. lemon scented
    d. peppermint scented

3. Room temperature for infant massage should be
    a. cool to stimulate activity
    b. at body temperature
    c. warm enough for a baby without clothes
    d. warm enough for the giver's comfort

4. The infant's emotional and social development is promoted during massage by
    a. very light touch
    b. eye contact and talking
    c. joint movements
    d. soft towel placed underneath

5. The pressure used for infant massage should be
    a. penetrating
    b. as light as possible
    c. enough to cause reddening
    d. firm yet gentle

6. List the benefits of massage for infants.

20. MASSAGE FOR THE ELDERLY

1. As a healthy aging strategy, massage should be received
   a. sporadically
   b. regularly
   c. intermittently
   d. once a year

2. Massage slows the aging process by reducing
   a. blood and lymph circulation
   b. muscle contraction
   c. nerve conduction
   d. negative effects of stress

3. Joint mobilizations and stretching are especially useful for
   a. increasing circulation
   b. improving mobility
   c. enhancing mental alertness
   d. moisturizing skin

4. Avoid this movement when massaging the elderly:
   a. hyperextension of the neck
   b. hamstring stretch
   c. mobilizing techniques for the ankle
   d. mobilizing techniques for the shoulder

5. To improve the pliability of tissues in the elderly, use
   a. vibration techniques
   b. lots of oil
   c. petrissage techniques
   d. deep friction

7. List important cautions when giving massage to the elderly.

8. Describe the general goals for massage for healthy aging.

21. MASSAGE FOR THE TERMINALLY ILL AND DYING

1. That massage can contribute to the wellbeing of the terminally ill is
   a. impossible
   b. a contradiction
   c. a wellness perspective
   d. an optimist's dream

2. Massage techniques for the terminally ill are
   a. complex and advanced
   b. basic and simple
   c. specialized and advanced
   d. focused on cure

3. The length of massage sessions for the seriously ill is typically
   a. 20 minutes
   b. 60 minutes

c. 90 minutes
d. 120 minutes

4. Nonprofessional caregivers of the terminally ill can easily learn to give
   a. Abdominal massage
   b. Neck massage
   c. Hand and arm massage
   d. Full-body relaxation massage

5. A unique form of communication provided by massage is
   a. verbal
   b. written
   c. nonverbal
   d. telepathic

6. List special benefits of massage for inactive or bedridden terminally ill persons.

7. Identify emotional and social benefits of massage that contribute to the well-being of the terminally ill.

8. List benefits of massage for the inactive and bedridden person.

22. SEATED MASSAGE IN THE WORKPLACE

1. Seated massage in the workplace is focused on the
   a. hands and feet
   b. abdomen and chest
   c. lower body
   d. upper body

2. Seated massage for the workplace typically lasts for
   a. 5–6 minutes
   b. 10–20 minutes
   c. 30–40 minutes
   d. 50–60 minutes

3. To position the recipient correctly for seated massage,
   a. adjust the massage chair to fit his or her body
   b. have the recipient move to fit the chair
   c. talk the recipient through adjusting the chair themselves
   d. no positioning necessary

4. Good body mechanics for giving seated massage includes using
   a. straight leg stance leaning forward
   b. horse stance leaning forward
   c. deep lunging stance
   d. deep knee bend stance

5. Good techniques to use on the head and scalp are
   a. deep friction and hacking tapotement
   b. kneading and vibration
   c. circular friction and tapping tapotement
   d. effleurage and vibration

6. Describe the benefits of seated massage in the workplace.

7. List the techniques typically used for seated massage.

Video Segment Answer Key

1. BODY MECHANICS

1. To determine proper table height, stand at the side of the table with hands hanging down. The table should be at your
   c. first or second knuckles

2. Lower your body by bending at the
   b. knees

3. Apply pressure by
   a. shifting the weight

4. The wrist should be kept in this position as much as possible to avoid strain.
   c. neutral

5. To avoid strain when applying thumb pressure, be sure that thumb and wrist joints are
   d. in straight alignment

6. During compression techniques, the reinforcing hand is placed over the bottom hand's
   b. metacarpals

7. Proper body mechanics while sitting include keeping the head over the shoulders and the back in good alignment, sitting near the edge of the chair with the feet flat on the floor, and adjusting the chair to a height that allows good mechanics.

8. Two stances to use while performing massage are the front leaning stance or lunge and the horse stance.

2. POSITIONING AND DRAPING

1. When the recipient is supine, place bolsters
   b. under the knees and neck

2. When the recipient is prone, place bolsters
   c. under the ankles and shoulders

3. When a recipient is in side-lying position, place bolsters
   a. under the head, bent upper leg, and upper arm

4. The genitals and women's breasts are
   c. draped at all times

5. The technique used to secure the drape when the recipient is turning over is called
   b. tenting

6. The purposes of good draping include to ensure the recipient's modesty, comfort, and safety and to facilitate the smooth application of techniques.

7. The guidelines for good draping include providing a sheet or towel that is thick and large enough; covering genitals and women's breasts at all times; covering the body part to be massaged and then covering it again when finished; and tucking the drape to secure it.

3. INTRODUCTION TO WESTERN MASSAGE

1. Match the following Western massage techniques with the descriptions below.
   a. effleurage—sliding
   b. petrissage—kneading
   c. friction—rubbing together
   d. tapotement—percussion
   e. vibration—trembling
   f. touch without movement—holding

4. EFFLEURAGE

1. Effleurage techniques are strokes that
   d. slide and glide

2. The pressure used for effleurage techniques should
   b. begin light and gradually deepen

3. The amount of oil used for effleurage should be
   c. limited to what is necessary

4. For body areas with dry skin or a lot of hair, the amount of oil used should be
   a. increased to avoid pulling

5. Deep effleurage is best applied to broad areas like the back using the
   d. forearm

6. The uses of effleurage techniques during massage include applying oil, warming an area, assessing the condition of tissues, connecting and transitioning, beginning or ending massage of an area, and accustoming the recipient to touch.

7. The general effects of effleurage techniques include increased circulation, general relaxation, and stretching the skin.

5. PETRISSAGE

1. Petrissage techniques
   c. lift or compress

2. The oil or lotion used for petrissage techniques should be
   d. minimal and light

3. Bruising and pinching may result from using
   a. too much pressure
4. When performing compression with the palms of the hands, avoid
   c. hyperextending the wrists
5. Skin rolling involves
   b. lifting the skin from tissues underneath
6. The effects of petrissage techniques include milking muscles of waste products; increasing local circulation; separating tissues; promoting muscular relaxation.
7. When applying petrissage techniques, use one or two hands depending on the size and shape of the body part being massaged; use little or no oil to prevent slipping; and use petrissage when the recipient is clothed.

6. FRICTION

1. Superficial friction causes
   b. warming of skin tissues
2. To prevent chaffing during superficial friction, be careful of
   c. the amount of pressure used
3. During deep friction techniques, the fingers should not
   a. slide over the skin
4. In applying Cyriax friction to a sheathed tendon, the tendon should be
   c. on maximum stretch
5. Before and/or after Cyriax friction use this modality on the site.
   a. ice
6. Three directions for applying deep friction techniques are transverse or across the direction of the fibers; parallel to the direction of fibers; and circular.
7. The desired effects for deep transverse or Cyriax friction are separation of tissue fibers and hyperemia or increased local circulation.

7. TAPOTEMENT

1. Tapotement techniques are also known as
   b. percussion
2. The proper application of tapotement is best described as
   d. light, rapid, rhythmic
3. Variations of tapotement are created by
   a. using different parts of the hands
4. A variation of tapotement used to treat lung congestion is
   c. cupping
5. A variation of tapotement appropriate for use on the head is
   a. tapping
6. Tapotement techniques are used during massage as a finishing technique for an area such as the back, legs, or head; or to end the massage session overall.
7. The major effect of tapotement techniques is stimulation of the nerve endings.

8. VIBRATION

1. Fine vibration is performed manually
   c. over a small area with the fingertips
2. Fine vibration is generated by the practitioner using tension in the
   a. forearms
3. Fine vibration over the abdomen is used
   b. to stimulate digestion and elimination
4. A type of coarse vibration involving joint movement as muscles of a limb are tossed from hand to hand is
   c. jostling
5. A form of coarse vibration used to relieve tension in an individual muscle is
   a. shaking
6. A professional electronic massager should have variable speeds and allow for both subtle and more vigorous movement.
7. The physiological effects of fine vibration include the stimulation of nerves and physiological processes such as digestion and elimination; while coarse relieves tension and helps relax muscles and muscle groups.

9. TOUCH WITHOUT MOVEMENT

1. Touch without movement may be described as
   c. skilled touch with specific therapeutic intention
2. Passive touch and holding are used during massage for
   b. calming and integration
3. An example of touch without movement used as a finishing technique on a supine recipient is
   c. holding the feet
4. During massage, touch without movement is used for providing a moment of calm and integration: for inducing calm, balancing energy, and imparting heat; and for ending the session.
5. At the end of a massage session when the recipient is supine, holding of the head and/or feet is commonly used; or if prone, passive touch to the back on the shoulder blades may be applied.

10. JOINT MOVEMENTS

1. Mobilizing techniques involve the free movement of joints
   c. well within their normal range
2. Mobilizing techniques can be described as
   a. free, loose, smooth
3. Stretching techniques involve
   b. elongating soft tissues around a joint
4. Before stretching, perform the following for best results:
   c. warm surrounding soft tissues
5. The following movements are *not* within the scope of massage therapy:
   c. forced joint movements beyond normal range

6. The potential effects of joint movements include stretching surrounding soft tissues, increasing flexibility, stimulating the production of synovial fluid, heightening kinesthetic awareness, inducing muscle relaxation, and helping recipients release unconscious muscle tension.

7. For safe joint movement applications, keep the movements within a comfortable normal range; keep the quality of mobilizing movements free and loose; use caution around abnormal or diseased joints; avoid movement of inflamed joints; and listen to recipient feedback.

11. MYOFASCIAL MASSAGE

1. The goal of myofascial massage is to
   c. separate adhering fascial tissues
2. An important principle of performance in myofascial massage is to
   b. enter the tissues slowly
3. Once the desired depth of penetration is reached, tissues are stretched
   d. horizontally
4. Tissues are stretched slowly until you feel
   b. a point of resistance
5. Hold the stretch of tissues until you feel
   b. a giving or elongation of tissues
6. The goals of myofascial massage are to separate fascial tissues that are adhering to each other and to soften rigid connective tissue.
7. Health problems caused by adhering myofascial tissues include limited mobility, postural distortion, and poor cellular nutrition.

12. NEUROMUSCULAR THERAPY

1. To the practitioner, trigger points feel like
   b. taut bands of tissue
2. When pressed, active trigger points refer pain to their
   d. reference zone
3. Trigger points are deactivated using a manual technique called
   a. ischemic compression
4. Trigger points are located by palpation *and*
   c. feedback from recipient
5. When a trigger point deactivates, the practitioner will feel
   b. softening of tissues
6. The negative effects of active trigger points include reduced flexibility, weakened muscles, and pain.
7. Common causes of trigger points include trauma, poor posture, repetitive strain, and overwork of muscles and tendons.

13. LYMPHATIC DRAINAGE MASSAGE

1. Lymphatic massage techniques are
   b. slow, light, repetitive

2. Lymphatic massage techniques cause the flow of intercellular fluid into
   d. lymph capillaries

3. The pressure used when performing lymphatic massage should be
   a. just enough to move the skin

4. In lymphatic massage, the direction of movement for each technique is toward
   c. the targeted lymph node

5. This performance error will close off the lymph capillaries:
   c. using too heavy pressure

6. Lymphatic massage improves the function of the lymphatic system through the mechanical displacement of lymph fluid and the substances it carries. This increases flow or circulation within the system.

14. REFLEXOLOGY

1. Pressure on specific spots on the feet is thought to stimulate
   d. corresponding areas in other parts of the body

2. Reflexology techniques and charts were developed in the 1940s by
   b. Eunice Ingham

3. This technique is used to press points systematically and quickly.
   c. thumb walking

4. This technique is used for deep pressure to a specific spot.
   a. hook and backup

5. Physiological effects of reflexology include normalizing tissues and improving function in the corresponding areas; increasing circulation in the feet and corresponding areas and organs; and promoting general relaxation.

15. POLARITY THERAPY

1. The goal of polarity therapy is to
   c. remove obstructions to energy flow

2. Many of the beneficial physiological effects of polarity therapy can be traced to
   b. mind and body relaxation

3. Polarity therapy can be described as
   a. simple touch and gentle movements

4. Major polarity therapy techniques are
   a. rocking, direct pressure, touch without movement

5. Each polarity therapy technique is held or performed for
   c. 1–2 minutes

16. ACUPRESSURE TECHNIQUE

1. The intent of Asian bodywork is to
   b. facilitate the flow of chi

2. The four pillars of assessment in Asian bodywork are
   d. seeing, touching, hearing/smelling, asking

3. For good body mechanics when performing Asian bodywork on a massage table, set the table height
   b. lower than Western massage

4. In Asian bodywork, pressure is applied to acupoints using
   a. weight transfer

5. The correct angle of penetration of acupoints is
   c. 90 degrees

6. Four principles of good body mechanics for applying pressure to acupoints are weight transfer, perpendicular penetration (90 degrees), stacking the joints, and proper alignment of the back and neck.

17. SPORTS MASSAGE

1. The primary goal of pre-event sports massage is
   c. readiness

2. Pre-event massage can be described as
   a. upbeat, short, fast paced

3. The primary goal of postevent massage is
   c. recovery

4. This technique is *not* used in postevent massage:
   d. percussion

5. The pressure used in postevent massage is
   c. lighter than pre-event massage

6. The desired effects for pre-event massage include increased circulation, warm muscles, ease of movement, and increased mental clarity and focus.

7. In determining whether an athlete is ready for postevent massage, be sure that he or she is cooled down, has taken adequate fluids, and is breathing normally.

18. PREGNANCY MASSAGE

1. Pregnancy massage is
   b. gentle and relaxing

2. Typical pregnancy posture causes strain in the
   c. lower back

3. The arms and legs of pregnant women are commonly
   a. swollen

4. Avoid massage of this area in pregnant women
   b. abdomen

5. The benefits of massage for pregnant women include general relaxation; release of emotional stress caused by hormonal changes and changing life circumstances; relief of physical stress in lower back, legs, and feet; reduced swelling in the extremities.

6. For pregnant women in the side-lying position bolsters are placed under the head, upper arm, upper leg, under the belly, and wherever else they are needed for comfort and support.

7. Contraindications for pregnancy massage include morning sickness and nausea; fever; vaginal bleeding or discharge; decreased fetal movement; diarrhea; pain in the abdomen; and excessive swelling of the arms or legs.

19. INFANT MASSAGE

1. Massage helps the development of a baby's nervous system through
   c. tactile stimulation and movement
2. The oil used for infant massage should be
   a. unscented
3. Room temperature for infant massage should be
   c. warm enough for a baby without clothes
4. The infant's emotional and social development is promoted during massage by
   b. eye contact and talking
5. The pressure used for infant massage should be
   d. firm yet gentle
6. The benefits of massage for infants include relieving tension, learning to relax, improving sleep, assisting digestion and elimination, bonding with parents and caregivers, and calming colicky babies.

20. MASSAGE FOR THE ELDERLY

1. As a healthy aging strategy, massage should be received
   b. regularly
2. Massage slows the aging process by reducing
   d. negative effects of stress
3. Joint mobilizations and stretching are especially useful for
   b. improving mobility
4. Avoid this movement when massaging the elderly:
   a. hyperextension of the neck
5. To improve the pliability of tissues in the elderly, use
   c. petrissage techniques
6. Important cautions when giving massage to the elderly include modifying pressure; avoiding massage over varicose veins and on the lateral neck; not putting the neck in hyperextension; watching for skin cancer and lesions; and taking medications into consideration.
8. General goals for massage for healthy aging include moisturizing skin; improving circulation; relaxing muscles; increasing tissue pliability; improving mobility and posture; enhancing digestion and elimination; and providing social contact.

21. MASSAGE FOR THE TERMINALLY ILL AND DYING

1. That massage can contribute to the well-being of the terminally ill is
   c. a wellness perspective

2. Massage techniques for the terminally ill are
   b. basic and simple

3. The length of massage sessions for the seriously ill is typically
   a. 20 minutes

4. Nonprofessional caregivers of the terminally ill can easily learn to give
   c. Hand and arm massage

5. A unique form of communication provided by massage is
   c. nonverbal

6. Special benefits of massage for inactive or bedridden terminally ill persons include relief from insomnia, constipation, breathing difficulty and skin degeneration, plus improved digestion and elimination.

7. Emotional and social benefits of massage that contribute to the well-being of the terminally ill include reduced anxiety and depression, lessened sense of isolation, increased sense of well-being.

22. SEATED MASSAGE IN THE WORKPLACE

1. Seated massage in the workplace is focused on the
   d. upper body

2. Seated massage for the workplace typically lasts for
   b. 10–20 minutes

3. To position the recipient correctly for seated massage,
   a. adjust the massage chair to fit his or her body

4. Good body mechanics for giving seated massage includes using
   c. deep lunging stance

5. Good techniques to use on the head and scalp are
   c. circular friction and tapping tapotement

6. The benefits of seated massage in the workplace include stress reduction, increased mental clarity, alleviation of aches and pains from sitting or standing at a workstation, relief of tension headache, revitalization, and readiness to get back to work.

7. Techniques typically used for seated massage include those that can be applied easily over clothing such as compression, direct pressure, friction, kneading, and joint movements.